I Love You Always

I Love You Always

*One Family's Alzheimer's/Dementia Journey
and the Lessons Learned Along the Way*

LaBena Fleming

Contact LaBena Fleming: labenafleming.com

Independently Published 2020 through Kindle Direct Publishing.

Printed in the United States of America

Paperback ISBN: 9798655405752

Cover design by SelfPubBookCovers.com/RLSather

Edited by Blue Hyphen Creative, LLC

Note to the readers: This book has been written based upon my personal knowledge, experiences, and opinions. Because I am not a legal or medical professional, nor a dementia expert, I am not tendering legal, medical, or professional advice. Such services should be sought from professionals in the fields of the services and advice you seek.

Names of hospitals (with the exception of Cleveland Clinic), nursing homes, skilled nursing facilities and their staff are fictitious in nature and any resemblance to actual companies is entirely coincidental. Names of characters, with the exceptions of Lottie, Nettie, John, John III, are fictitious as well. Names of other organizations and businesses are being used with permission.

To My God

Lord, I hear your voice continuing to guide me. In the stillness of the night, when the pain comes, you comfort me. During the trials of the day, I feel your presence and know that you are close at hand. When I am weak, you strengthen me. When I feel I can't go on, you pour your love into me and let me know that I can do anything as long as I continue to lean on you. Thank you for being my help. I couldn't have survived this journey without you.

To My Mom

It was my honor to have been your daughter and to have been able to help care for you. It wasn't always easy, but there were many blessings along the way. Rest well. I miss you, and I love you always.

Honour thy father and thy mother: that thy days may be long upon the land which the Lord thy God giveth thee. Exodus 20:12

Contents

Foreword

I am a registered nurse who has been involved in the care of patients who have Alzheimer's disease and their families for many years. LaBena attended many of my lectures on Alzheimer's disease and generously shared her experiences of caring for her mother, who had Alzheimer's and vascular dementia. When she shared that she was writing a book, I felt confident it would be written with love and passion, but it far exceeded my expectations.

What I liked most about LaBena's book was the manner in which she shared her story of caring for her mother, baring her heart and soul. Her journey was not one that anyone chooses, and she and her family embarked on it knowing how it would end. What they didn't know was the magnitude of the peaks and valleys that would occur during the course of that journey. Through her words, LaBena was able to capture the depth of emotions that people experience when caring for a loved one who has dementia and share what she learned along the way.

The title, *I Love You Always*, is very fitting as she and her family showed the love they had for their mother throughout the challenging situations that presented themselves. LaBena's book is a must read for people embarking on this caregiver journey. You are not alone, and you will realize that, in spite of your situation, you can love always.

Linda Bliss, RN

Preface

I am no one special. I am simply the daughter of a mother who was diagnosed with dementia. I'd had the privilege of working with a hospice provider for several years prior to my mom's diagnosis, and it was during that time that I learned about dementia.

Sitting in our team meetings, I would hear about disease progression, caregiver tips, etc., and I was afforded the opportunity to receive special training on the basics of dementia that prepared me to educate community members who were caring for loved ones with the disease. Once I began caring for my mom, however, everything I thought I knew went right out of the window. It's one thing to learn about dementia, but it's totally different when you live it.

This book holds my truth: the good, the bad, and the ugly. My prayer is that you will be able to learn from my experiences, that you will look for light in the darkness, and that you will see and take advantage of the beautiful moments that present themselves during the journey. More importantly, I pray that you hold on to faith. It is faith that sustained me when I felt I couldn't go on for one more moment. God didn't promise that we wouldn't go through storms, but we can find comfort in knowing that He is right there with us through it all.

I can do all things through Christ which strengtheneth me.
Philippians 4:13

Author's note: All biblical quotations are from the King James Version of the Bible.

Acknowledgments

My husband, for sharing so unselfishly and for always being my rock.

My brothers, for being able to put Mom's needs ahead of your own and for working as a team.

My daughters and granddaughter, for brightening so many of Mom's days.

Hospice of the Western Reserve, for your exemplary education/training and care.

Crossroads Hospice, for being there and providing phenomenal care whenever we needed you.

Alzheimer's Association, for being a great resource for patients and their families.

Linda Bliss, RN, for your valuable education and training sessions.

National Council of Certified Dementia Practitioners, (NCCDP) for recognizing the importance of specialized training for those who work with persons who have dementia.

Caregivers, because you are so undervalued. Thanks for all you do.

Dementia Through Daughters Eyes Facebook Group, for your support.

#AMWRITING, especially Abby Vandiver, for encouraging me to just write my story.

Dr. Elizabeth C. Blackman, for your valuable insight and suggestions.

People with Alzheimer's and other forms of dementia, for your courage and your fire. May there soon be a cure.

A special thank you to all my friends who took the time to read and provide honest feedback on my manuscript. I love you!

Chapter 1
Before

I have always believed that God has an interesting sense of humor, and anyone who knew the story of my life would understand why. I just wondered whether today would be a day where He'd display that humor, and whether it would be cool, keen, or downright mean. Time would tell.

It's funny, the thoughts that enter a sleep-deprived mind. How ironic that *this* Easter Sunday, one of the holiest of holy days, would fall on April Fools' Day in 2018. I was not in the mood for jokes. I wasn't in the mood for anything other than sleep.

I laid awake listening to the ticking of my husband George's classic car wall clock and tried to slow down the thumping of my heart. It seemed to pound harder and louder with each beat, as if it would burst out of my chest any moment. Then that darned horn blew . . . the clock's way of letting me know that another hour had passed.

It was 6:00 a.m. and I was trying to lull myself to sleep. Sleep? It had eluded me for weeks, so I didn't know why I expected things to be different now. There was far too much chatter going on in my mind to allow me to rest. I'd sleep for only a few minutes here and there—or at most a couple of hours—grateful for whatever rest would find me. How I wished for more, but that wish was in vain.

Thoughts of my mom, Lottie Mae Polk Berry—who had been battling Alzheimer's and vascular dementia for years, and who was now fighting for her life—were flooding my mind. Mom, a self-proclaimed badass, was fierce and proud. She had more strength and tenacity than anyone I'd ever known. She loved hard and fought even harder for whatever—or whomever—she wanted, and what she believed in.

When I asked Mom a year ago if there was anything she had a desire to do, or anyone she wanted to see, she responded that she just wanted to live to see her ninetieth birthday. Although she never articulated why

1

it was so important to her, I deduced it was because no one else in her family had lived beyond their eighties. I never found any information contrary to that belief.

At that time, I was sure that her desire to live to ninety was a real possibility; however, I didn't feel that same certainty now. Would she be able to hold on for eighteen more hours?

I'd been praying hard and suspected that my brothers—even the ones who claimed not to believe in the power of prayer—were doing the same. I begged God to grant this last wish for Mom. It wasn't too much to ask of Him, was it?

I tried the old bargaining game: "God, if you allow Mom to live to see ninety, I'll be a better Christian. I'll become more involved in church and attend more regularly." I felt I'd been a good Christian and a dutiful daughter. My brothers and I worked hard to ensure that Mom's needs were being met. Surely, we could petition for her big wish as well! "God, please don't let this be *the* day."

And in that day ye shall ask me nothing. Verily, verily, I say unto you, whatsoever ye shall ask the Father in my name, He will give it to you. John 16:23

It was now 7:00 a.m., and I couldn't discern whether time was moving too slowly or too rapidly. I was exhausted and still not ready to get out of bed. Subconsciously, I began to reflect not only on this past year but also on Mom's life in general.

Mom was born on April 2, 1928 to Albert and Will Ella Polk in Bentonia, Mississippi. By all accounts, she had been a real pistol while growing up. She pretty much did what she wanted and accepted the punishments that would be doled out as a result.

As a teen, she was infamous for ordering things out of mail-order catalogs without permission and charging them to her father. She would also go to the general store in town and purchase items using her dad's credit account, knowing she would be punished later. When I questioned why she had done such things, her response was, "The spankings I'd get would only hurt for a little while, but I always got to keep the stuff." That was badass indeed!

Her cousin Nina, who was raised by my grandparents, had told me that Mom liked to pick fights and cause trouble. "She wasn't happy unless she was starting some mess," Nina told me. When I asked Mom why she behaved like that, she said, "Because it was fun. There was no fun in being good."

As if those challenges were not enough, it was in her teens that Mom met her future husband, John Willis Berry Jr., whose family had a farm nearby. According to Mom, their relationship caused my grandparents so much stress that they sent her away to boarding school in an attempt to keep the two of them apart.

By her own account, Mom was pure trouble while at boarding school, and my grandfather had to make frequent visits to convince the school to allow her to stay. Mom later shared that she was sure Grandpa and the headmistress "had a little something going on." In her mind, that was the only logical explanation for the school not kicking her out (which was her goal).

The tactic of sending Mom to boarding school did not accomplish the desired result of keeping her apart from my dad. Story has it that one day, out of the blue, Dad asked Mom if she wanted to get married. She said yes, and they immediately went to town and got married. None of their parents were pleased with the union, but the deed had been done. Perhaps their parents were able to see what Mom and Dad were unable to see: they were just not good together.

Their relationship was extremely tumultuous and, at times, violent. Mom took great pride in the fact that she could "dish it out as well as she could take it." Despite the constant battles and endless separations— or perhaps because of it—seven children were born into that union: Don, Lewis, John III, me, Daniel, Andrew, and Nicholas. My dad also had another son, Peter, from a relationship he'd had before marrying my mom. Mom and Dad eventually made their way to Ravenna, Ohio, where my siblings (except Peter) and I were raised.

I don't have many pleasant memories of Mom and Dad's time together, but I do remember how well they worked together when my brother, Andrew, was born. He was such a beautiful baby and I remember being a little jealous because he was so pretty. He had smooth, caramel-colored skin, deep cocoa-brown eyes, and coal-black eyelashes that almost reached his eyebrows when he closed his eyes. I was envious because, as the only daughter, I felt those looks should have been mine.

Although Andrew appeared perfect on the exterior, the coming months would reveal that he was far from perfect. A cancerous tumor was found on his spine. I can't remember surgeries or chemo, but I am fairly confident that he endured both. I can, however, remember the constant trips Mom and Dad made to the Cleveland Clinic for Andrew's treatments and care.

While at home, Andrew was showered with attention from all of us. I was four years older than him and viewed him as a doll. He loved the song "A Little Bit of Soap," which we always sang to him. I can still picture his beautiful smile. When Andrew was around, Mom and Dad didn't fight. The family functioned like a well-oiled machine. When Andrew was around, we all focused on him.

Unfortunately, Andrew lost his battle with cancer at the age of two. It was during his short life that I first witnessed the strength of my mother. Being a mother now myself, I can't begin to imagine how painful the experience of having a critically ill child—and later losing that child—could be. I don't think I could survive it, but she did.

I was only six when Andrew died, and I remember begging to go to his funeral. Initially, my parents thought I was too young and were concerned about the impact that attending a funeral would have on me. Eventually, they conceded to my relentless requests. It turned out to be a great benefit to me: as I saw my brother laying in the casket, it was the first time I saw him fully at peace. I understood that he was now pain-free and resting in the arms of God and the angels. Instead of remembering the pain he endured, I remember the vision of total calm as he lay in his casket.

We are confident, I say, and willing rather to be absent from the body, and to be present with the Lord. 2 Corinthians 5:8

I knew my mom and dad were grieving, but they never allowed us to see their grief. In the early 1960s, there were no hospice providers or grief support groups that we were aware of. We all dealt with the loss of Andrew in our own way, but Mom displayed an extraordinary strength. She didn't miss a beat in the way she cared for the rest of us, despite everything she was dealing with.

It would be many years before I would see and understand the toll that the experience had had on her. Although Andrew's illness and subsequent death were my first recollections of seeing how strong my mother was, unfortunately, they wouldn't be my last.

Chapter 2
The Struggle Is Real

The years that followed would have our family witness the good, the bad, and the ugly with regard to my parents' relationship. The fights continued and were becoming more violent. There would be many separations and reconciliations—and three divorces. Yes, they remarried twice! They loved hard but they fought harder.

I was relieved when they divorced because I didn't have to sleep with one eye open, listening to the magnitude of their fights and wondering if either one of them would make it out alive. By the same token, I was upset each time they reconciled because I knew, after the initial honeymoon phase, we'd end up right back where we started. The fighting and arguing would eventually resume and my anxiety and stress levels would be through the roof.

I know my dad was the love of Mom's life, but I always questioned his devotion to her. Although Dad's love of women was the reason behind many of their fights, Mom always forgave him. I have no recollection of her ever seeing another man during their times of separation; my dad, however, was a different story. He not only dated other women but ended up living with multiple women during their separations.

This hurt Mom to her core, but she never gave up on him. She never stopped loving him and never stopped her quest to get him back. Much to Mom's chagrin, their third marriage and subsequent divorce would mark the end of their relationship.

Dad seemed content with his new life and twenty-something girlfriend. Mom hung on to the idea of reconciliation until his death in 1985 at the age of fifty-nine. The pain she felt when he died was palpable. Although she remained strong, a huge piece of herself died when Dad died. She would never give her heart to another man.

Even though a large part of Mom and Dad's social life had revolved around alcohol, cigars, and cigarettes, it wasn't until Dad's death that I saw an increase in Mom's drinking. Whenever I'd question or challenge her, she would say that drinking helped her make it through the day. I began to see the toll her losses were taking on her.

I would recommend support groups and counseling to her, but she felt she was doing fine and didn't need any help. She'd always say, "If I want to stop drinking, I can stop drinking. I'm just fine so mind your own damn business."

I never labeled Mom as an alcoholic because she truly was able to stop drinking whenever she chose to do so. She loved the taste of beer and how she felt when she drank it. Alcohol—specifically, Miller High Life—was Mom's coping mechanism.

Mom was truly high functioning and controlled. She never missed work or any events because of her drinking. She only drank at home and, as I mentioned earlier, was able to stop for long periods of time if a situation warranted it. In her mind, Mom didn't need help and didn't want help. She loved beer, period!

Unfortunately, although she felt her drinking was not a problem, her children and grandchildren saw things differently. When Mom drank, she lacked a filter, always saying whatever came to mind regardless of the impact it would have on others. Her early years as a troublemaker followed her into her later years. Mom just didn't seem happy unless she was in some kind of mess.

I found myself constantly trying to defend Mom to my siblings and their spouses. Trying to play peacemaker became a painful part of my existence; it was mentally and emotionally draining. Although I loved my mom deeply and dearly, I did not like her when she was drinking. Neither did anyone else, and many of her loved ones began to disengage with her.

The mid-1990s would present new challenges for my mom. I can remember as if it were yesterday the day my coworker, Jerry, advised me that a call had come in stating that my mom had been taken to the hospital. I had been in the process of changing offices due to a promotion and had been away from my desk.

Jerry had no details about what had happened, but I got a bad feeling in the pit of my stomach and burst into tears. I don't know why I was crying, as I had no idea what had occurred. I just had a strong sense that whatever had happened was not good.

I remembered a dream I'd had about a month earlier. In the dream, Dad told me to be sure to take care of Mom because she needed me. I thought it was funny at the time because my mom was fiercely independent and would be highly insulted if someone attempted to take care of her. I had dismissed the dream as having no merit.

As I returned to my former department to get my purse and head to the hospital, tears streamed down my face. People who saw me crying thought I was emotional because it was my last day with them. They had no clue what was going on, and I wasn't about to take time to explain things to them. As I rushed out, I asked Jerry to please provide everyone with an explanation of what was happening. He agreed.

When I reached the hospital, I was greeted by my then five brothers: Don, Lewis, John III, Daniel, and Nicholas. I felt as if my heart was going to stop beating as they informed me that Mom had had a stroke and they were waiting to learn more from the doctors. As was my habit, I began my bargaining process with God. "If you let my mom live, I'll be a much better person, and I'll go to church more regularly . . . and I'll draw closer to you." Isn't it funny how we pull out our bargaining chips when we need something? I don't believe God bargains, but I was desperate.

After what seemed like hours, we were finally permitted to see Mom. We were pleasantly surprised when she recognized all of us; however, she seemed to be confused and having difficulty with her vision. Tests revealed that a stroke had occurred on the right side, directly behind her eye, which explained why she was having difficulty seeing. She was also experiencing weakness in her left arm. Inpatient therapy at a skilled nursing facility (SNF) was recommended.

Because my brother Daniel had been an aide in the physical therapy department where Mom was hospitalized, he was convinced he could do whatever therapy she needed at home. This greatly pleased her, as she had no interest in going to a nursing home for any reason.

My brothers and I decided to go to Mom's home to see what needed to be done to make it rehab friendly. Upon reaching her living room, I burst into tears again. The house looked like it had been hit by a tornado. Chairs were overturned. Papers were strewn all over, and there was evidence that Mom had attempted to bake John's and Daniel's birthday cakes on top of the stove instead of in the oven.

John, who discovered Mom when he came home for lunch, stated that water was running from every faucet in the house when he arrived and that all burners on the stove were on. Thank God he came home for lunch that day. I can only imagine what could have happened had he not done so.

While we were cleaning the house, I had a flashback to my dream of Dad telling me to take care of Mom. Little did I know at the time that the dream foreshadowed things to come.

We continued to put things in order to ensure a smooth transition when Mom came home. John agreed he would check in on her daily during his lunch breaks; the rest of us committed to coming by during the day as our work schedules permitted. Daniel would supplement the in-home therapy by working with her in the evenings when he got home from work.

Mom returned home and responded very well to her therapy sessions. In just a few weeks, except for a loss of math aptitude and some vision loss, Mom was pretty much back to her pre-stroke self.

Despite a successful recovery, Mom quickly became frustrated because she was losing some of her independence. She now had to rely on me for money management; her finances had always been her business. This was frustrating for me as well because Mom became obsessed with the idea that she might not have enough money to cover her monthly bills. She called me constantly. "How much money do I have in the bank? Did you pay the electric bill? John might be stealing my money. How much money did you say I have?"

I accepted those calls as our new normal and did what I needed to do. As I recognized how much worse everything could have been, I couldn't help but praise and thank God for this victory.

Mom was again showing her tremendous strength, fortitude, and determination. I was amazed by her resilience.

Mom gained back all of her physical strength after the stroke. Unfortunately, such was not the case with her mental and visual capabilities. She never regained her number sense, which meant I had become her forever money manager. Also, her personality had become more challenging since her stroke.

These things I have spoken unto you, that in me ye might have peace. In the world ye shall have tribulation: but be of good cheer; I have overcome the world. John 16:33

Chapter 3
Put to the Test

For the first few years following her stroke, Mom's condition held steady. Unfortunately, February 27, 2001, would present Mom with yet one more opportunity for her to display her strength.

While heading home from a class (I was then pursuing my elementary teaching certification), I had gone to the grocery store to pick up supplies for the chicken parmesan and rice pilaf that I planned to prepare for the family of a friend whose father had recently died. Those were the comfort foods I always took to the homes of bereaved friends. While in the store, I also searched for a sympathy card.

Buying cards has always been an arduous task for me because I am ritualistic about it. Everything about the card must be perfect. First, I preview the image on the cover to see what type of emotion it evokes, and then ask myself whether the words on the cover adequately convey my thoughts. Finally, I consider what my immediate thoughts were after reading the content.

When I had found a card at the grocery store that contained everything I had wanted to convey, I remember thinking, "This card would bring me comfort." How ironic that in just minutes, comforting would be exactly what I'd need.

I arrived home, unloaded my books and groceries, changed clothes, washed up, and began to prepare the meal to take to my friend's home. I prepared my secret chicken coating (a mixture of breadcrumbs, special seasonings, and parmesan cheese) and had just placed the freshly breaded chicken in the skillet when the phone rang. All of my friends knew how much I hated speaking on the phone and rarely called. As such, I never answered the phone; I don't know what caused me to answer it this time.

I heard Daniel's voice and immediately held my breath. Daniel always called my cell phone. The house phone, I'd come to learn, was reserved for bad news. I think he used the technique of calling the house phone with the hopes that my husband George would answer and be able to prepare me for the news to come.

When I heard Daniel utter the word, "Sis," I knew he was bearing bad news. Normally, he'd begin the conversation with, "How are you doing, sis?"

I don't know how long it took me to breathe and listen to what was being said. I recall hearing "John" and "heart attack" and being able to put together that John had had a heart attack while working out at the gym. I started to tell Daniel to let John know I was on my way when he interrupted, saying, "He didn't make it."

I fell to the floor . . . I think I may have briefly passed out. I could hear George talking but couldn't make sense of his words. I could also hear my daughter, Lynn, sobbing. I then realized that as much as I wanted it all to be a dream, it was real. John, my beloved brother, was dead at the young age of forty-six.

I had just spoken to him the previous Sunday. We had planned to get together, but I canceled our "date" because I needed to study. If I had kept it, perhaps I would have seen something was wrong and convinced him to seek medical attention. Perhaps I could have intervened in some way, I thought. Could I have saved him if I'd met with him? But it was not to be. I couldn't go back and change what had happened. John was gone, and there was absolutely nothing I could do about it.

As I began to regain my composure, I immediately thought of my mom and the fact that this would be the second son she would have to bury. First Andrew, and now John. A mom is not supposed to outlive her children! How was she going to handle this?

Mom had buried a loved one every decade since the 1960s when Andrew died. Her father died in 1974; my dad in 1985; her mother in 1994; and now John. She'd also managed to have a minor heart attack in 1975 (shortly after I'd married my first husband), and then the stroke.

I wondered when she would reach her breaking point. I also wondered when I would reach mine.

I needed to see my mom. I needed to see my brother. I needed to feel not so helpless. I needed strength. Lord, I need you now, I thought.

I quickly packed a bag because I knew I would be staying with Mom for a while. John had lived with her, so she would have quite an adjustment. Because he never married and had no children, Mom would be responsible for making the funeral arrangements. She was going to need me, and I was going to need her. It's odd to think that in 2001, she was mentally capable of making important decisions. How quickly things would change!

George insisted upon driving me from our home in Richmond Heights to Ravenna, and I didn't argue. I was in no condition to drive. Lynn accompanied us as well, after ensuring that the stove was turned off and things were in order. That was the longest hour-long drive I had ever experienced, although I'm sure it didn't take that long. Regardless, it felt like an eternity by the time we'd reached the hospital.

I raced through the emergency entrance, with George and Lynn following closely behind. I don't know why there was such a sense of urgency. John was gone and there was nothing anyone could do about it. I looked past my brothers—Don, Lewis, Daniel, and Nicholas—as I found my way to Mom. She looked into my eyes and said, "They killed my son!" I could not contain my sobs as I hugged her, and then followed Daniel to John's room.

He was so still. I hated that the intubation tube was protruding from his mouth. Why couldn't they remove that thing before we'd arrived? I touched him but he didn't touch me back. John always touched me back. Whenever he'd see me, he'd give me a big hug, kiss me, and tell me he loved me. He always told me, and showed me, that he loved me.

John would never be able to tell me he loved me again. He would never hug me again.

Mom and I worked together on the funeral arrangements for John. Our family was astounded by the outpouring of love and support we received from the community. John had been employed within the Juvenile Court System for years and had positively impacted many lives.

It was the support we received, and the love we were shown, that made the ordeal of John's death and subsequent burial more bearable. The food, calls, and cards we received—along with the stories we were told—showed us the extent of John's impact on the small Ravenna community. I watched Mom beam with pride at each story she heard and, I believe, she loved the attention she was receiving. She certainly didn't like the reason, but she relished the attention.

I believe it was that positive attention that fed her spirit during the difficult days and months that followed. Mom attended multiple functions and accepted many awards on John's behalf for more than a year following his death. But with that attention also came many challenges.

Mom's decision to show up at every event where he was being remembered or honored kept her from being able to move forward with her grief. In addition, she would soon have the major challenge of rectifying a prior act of kindness with the negative impact that followed.

A few years before John's death, Mom decided to put her home in John's and Daniel's names and award herself lifetime tenancy. This meant that, although the home was in John's and Daniel's names, she would be a lifelong resident of the home. She had done this because Don, Lewis, Nicholas, and I were all married and owned our own homes. Daniel and John were single, non-homeowners who devoted themselves to Mom. This was her way of thanking them for their commitment to her and ensuring they had a home when she died.

No one could have imagined that another of Mom's children would precede her in death, so her decision sounded like a good idea at the time. Unfortunately, John's heart was much bigger than his wallet. We learned he had often given to others, to the extent that he put himself in great debt. For the home to revert to Mom, she had to pay off John's debts. Otherwise, creditors would have gone after her home to receive payment.

Fortunately, John had listed Mom as the primary beneficiary on his life insurance. She was able to use that money to pay off his debts and regain ownership of her home. This was an extremely stressful time for Mom, and I was concerned about her physical and emotional health. True to form, she would again show her tremendous strength and resilience.

Lesson: When doing estate planning, make sure you are fully aware of the positive and negative implications of the decisions you make.

Chapter 4
A Change Is Gonna Come

There was no change in Mom's condition until a couple of years after John's death. She had managed to break her ankle after falling from a ladder, while wrestling with a damaged tree branch. This was unusual behavior for her, as she was not one to do outside work. Besides, Daniel and Lewis normally took care of all things outdoors.

The broken ankle seemed to send my mom into a downward spiral. After the break, she stopped going for daily walks at the Kent State University track, which she had done religiously in years prior. She also constantly complained of body aches and pain, which was not the norm for her.

Mom's primary care physician attributed everything to age and arthritis. Because of the doctor's comments, we weren't concerned until we began to see other changes. Mom was always tired and seemed weak. She was also showing signs of depression.

When these concerns were expressed to her physician, we were told this was a normal part of aging. Mom was now seventy-nine and we had never witnessed anyone living to that age. With all the losses she had experienced, and now that she was not doing tasks she had regularly done in the past, we also felt Mom's depression was normal.

But as her memory, mood, and depression became worse, I was no longer convinced that what she was experiencing was normal. I knew my mom and felt strongly that something just wasn't right. I put my detective hat on.

Upon reviewing Mom's recent blood work, I noticed she had high levels of calcium in her blood. When I added that to the fact that she'd been complaining of aches and pains, her weakness and fatigue, depression, and what appeared to be brittle bones (she had broken a toe since breaking her ankle), I was convinced that Mom suffered from hyperparathyroidism. According to Mayoclinic.org, "Hyperparathyroidism is an excess of parathyroid hormones in the bloodstream due to over activity of one or more of the body's four parathyroid glands."

I bombarded my siblings with information I copied from various websites regarding hyperparathyroidism. The siblings who'd taken time to review the information agreed that hyperparathyroidism looked like a real possibility.

I then found an endocrinologist who would either confirm or dispel my diagnosis. After Mom completed a battery of tests, we learned that she did indeed have a parathyroid disorder. Parathyroid glands are part of the endocrine system. According to Parathyroid.com, "[Parathyroid glands] are small, and their role is to control the amount of calcium in our bones and blood." If they are not functioning properly, a host of physical and psychological problems can result.

The recommended treatment for hyperparathyroidism is surgery. The first specialist we visited suggested that we do nothing due to Mom's age; there were no guarantees her mental state would improve after surgery. A second specialist, however, felt that we could see a marked improvement in Mom's condition if she had the surgery

Imaging tests showed enlargement of all four parathyroid glands, but no tumors. The plan was to remove three of the four glands and remove a portion of the fourth, relocating the remaining portion to Mom's wrist. Hoping for a remedy for her symptoms, we all agreed to the surgery.

My brothers and I were present for the surgery and we were beyond hopeful. Thank God, the surgery went very well. Mom was pleasant when she awakened, and we were told that any behavioral changes would be gradual. The endocrinologist advised us, "It will take time for everything that has been malfunctioning to correct itself." Unfortunately, over time, there were no improvements in Mom's condition. In fact, we began to see more negative changes.

We came to learn that surgery can have very negative consequences for the elderly. Mom's short-term memory and reasoning skills became worse after surgery. Neither of the two specialists had discussed those negative possibilities with us when we spoke of the pros and cons of surgery. I didn't understand that.

Perhaps that's why the first specialist did not feel that the surgery should be done. Why didn't he tell us that? Did he tell us that and we weren't listening? Were we just so hell-bent on a cure that we didn't hear his rationale for not wanting to perform surgery on Mom?

I felt that the increase in the negative symptoms were my fault, and I experienced tremendous guilt for having had her go through an unnecessary surgery. I was the one who had gone searching for other causes of her behaviors. I was the one who had provided my brothers with information that caused them to hope for a cure.

I wondered if my brothers were secretly angry with me but didn't dare ask. That surgery became the elephant in the room. We never spoke of it, just like we never spoke about what could really be going on with Mom.

Over the next year, we witnessed quite a few physical and cognitive changes in Mom. We always reverted to her physician's saying that it was all a normal part of aging. Although we felt that what we were seeing was more than normal aging, we didn't challenge what we were being told.

Lesson: If you have a strong sense that something is wrong, something probably is wrong—and it won't just go away.

As 2007 drew to a close, we were forced to look back upon the troubling things that had occurred in the recent past. Why had those unexplainable dings and dents appeared on Mom's car? Why was she forgetful and argumentative? Why was she so accusatory? Why was she making up romances/relationships for various siblings? Why did she think everyone was stealing from her? Why was she constantly losing or misplacing things?

Since I had served as a provider relations manager with Hospice of the Western Reserve (HWR) for many years and had facilitated countless community and professional education sessions on the basics of dementia, I had a good understanding of what the signs and symptoms were. I was just choosing to be in denial, so I wouldn't have to face the reality of what was to be. I wouldn't have to begin the grieving process, knowing that I would lose my mom bit by bit. I could pretend that everything going on with Mom was just a normal part of aging.

Because of my experience with the hyperparathyroidism diagnosis, there was no way I was going to share my suspicions with my siblings this time. I was determined to let Mom's physician do her job. I began accompanying her to appointments to share what I was seeing and hear what the doctor had to say.

At this point in time, there had been no mention of dementia, and I was darned if I was going to be the first person to bring it up. I would just continue to watch, wait, and document.

Lesson: What I have learned is that we sometimes find comfort in not knowing. When we deny something exists, we don't have to deal with it. We don't have to anticipate or plan. We don't have to stress about it. We don't have to do anything . . . until we have to.

Chapter 5
2008: It Will Be All Right

Daniel said, "Sis . . . " I sucked in my breath, and tears began to immediately well up in my eyes. What relief I'd felt this time when he told me to breathe and said that no one had died. I wondered if he heard my sigh of relief as he told me that Mom had fallen and that he'd called an ambulance because he was unable to lift her.

I found that quite odd. Mom was a slight woman, barely five feet two and just shy of 125 pounds. Daniel, on the other hand, was five feet eleven and weighed over two hundred pounds. He worked in a hospital and lifted people all day. Why was he unable to lift her? As if reading my thoughts, he told me that it was like trying to lift dead weight.

My mind was racing. Although Daniel suggested that I not come to Ravenna until he knew what was going on, he knew better. If Mom was going to the hospital, I would be there.

As the only daughter, I'd learned that brothers think very differently. With me, emotion always came into play when dealing with situations, but such was not the case with my brothers. Most times, everything was matter-of-fact with them. I guess that's why Daniel hadn't felt the need for me to come to Ravenna until he knew more.

Mom fell. Daniel couldn't lift her. She was within two feet of the telephone—yet she didn't call him for help—and he didn't see a need for me to come? RIGHT!

I quickly put some overnight things together, told George what was going on, and headed to Ravenna. George wanted to drive me, but I didn't want to wait for him to finish what he was doing. Although Daniel had stated there was no urgency, I needed to leave immediately.

I recall getting into my car and being more stressed than I thought I'd be. I didn't know what was going on with Mom, and many thoughts flooded my mind: God, please keep me focused and safe on my drive—

and please don't take my mom. I was probably being melodramatic, but it was my mom!

I arrived at the hospital in about forty-five minutes, but it seemed like hours. When I reached the emergency room, Don, Lewis, Daniel, and Nicholas stood to greet me. I froze as I reflected on the last time that scene had presented itself to me, when John had died. I snapped back to the present. This time, everyone was smiling. I could breathe! Daniel said, "I told you not to come, but I knew you would." He knew me well! There was no way I was going to take anyone's word about how my mom was doing. I had to see her for myself. She would be expecting me.

Once I was permitted, I went to Mom's room, gave her a big hug, and asked how she was feeling. She told me she was fine and that there was nothing wrong. She just wanted to go home, she said. She was unable to tell me how she'd landed on the floor, but she did recall being unable to get up. When I asked why she hadn't used the phone to call for help, she said it was because she knew that Daniel, who lived in a mobile home on her property, was on his way. She decided that she would just wait for him. She wasn't in any pain and was fine. I knew she wasn't fine.

Mom was unable to walk, so a series of tests were run while in the emergency room. The doctors decided to keep her for observation. A CT scan of her spine had shown that she had severe spinal stenosis, which, according to Wikipedia, is "an abnormal narrowing of the spinal canal or neural foramen that results in pressure on the spinal cord or nerve roots." According to the physicians, this caused weakness in her legs and impeded her ability to walk.

Lesson: Being admitted under observation is not the same as a regular hospital admittance and could impact if/how your hospital stay is paid. It can also determine whether Medicare will cover any portion of a subsequent stay at a skilled nursing facility (SNF) for rehabilitation. Be sure to have a case manager explain what the impact of being admitted under observation will have on costs and the billing process.

Surgery was not an option as far as we were concerned because we'd learned our lesson with our last experience. Since Mom was eighty years of age, we were not willing to take the risks associated with surgery. Instead, the recommended option was to have her go for rehabilitative therapy at a SNF. The goal was to strengthen her to the point that she would be able to walk and return home, which was her desire.

But Mom was not at all thrilled at the idea of being away from her home, and she made sure everyone knew it. What was disconcerting to all of us were the problems that surfaced while she was in the hospital. She kept forgetting where she was and became extremely upset and agitated when the hospital staff entered her room, which she thought was her home. Although Mom had been experiencing confusion for quite some time, this level of confusion was new and distressing to her—and to us.

It was time for us to pick a SNF, but there weren't many in Ravenna and we didn't know of anyone who had used the few that were in existence. We finally decided upon Cedar Glen, which was located close to Central Hospital, where Daniel was working. Because he was deemed legally blind at an early age and did not drive, this would make it easier for him to visit Mom. Location was not an issue for the rest of us.

After spending a couple of nights under observation in the hospital, Mom was moved to Cedar Glen. I think everyone, except Mom, was happy that she would be in a place where she would be closely monitored and taken care of. Daniel would be given a much-needed break, and the rest of us would know she was receiving good care . . .

or so we assumed. Mom, on the other hand, was livid. Even though she was still unable to walk, she wanted to go home. There was no rationalizing with her. She wanted to be at home, in her bed, and that was that. However, that was not possible.

We had no idea of the challenges to come, but we would soon be forced to face that which we had been in denial of for quite some time.

The Lord is my portion, saith my soul; therefore I will hope in him. Lamentations 3:24

Chapter 6
Rehab: Round One

Day one of rehab was interesting, to say the least. Although Mom fussed and complained about everything, her desire to go home ensured her compliance with the physical therapists. She knew she couldn't go home if she was unable to walk, and she knew she wouldn't be able to walk without physical therapy.

To ensure someone was with her as often as possible, my brothers and I adjusted and juggled our schedules to the best of our abilities. The SNF staff frequently commented on how devoted we were and wished all families of patients were like ours. I smirked each time I heard those words. I knew we were visible now but was concerned about what would happen once Mom went home. I knew us!

Shortly after her admittance to Cedar Glen, the staff had to remove the phone from Mom's room because—just as she had attempted to do in the hospital—she kept calling the police. She thought she was in her home and that strangers were coming in uninvited. The police came to the facility at one point, but upon realizing how confused Mom was, did not return. Red flags continued to appear. Her behavior was becoming stranger and we needed answers.

My brothers and I decided to have a conversation with Mom's attending physician at the SNF and insisted upon an MRI or CT scan of her brain. This was basically a formality; we all had a pretty good idea of what was going on. Mom was showing signs of dementia, but we wanted to rule out other possible reasons for her behavior.

Through my prior work experience and training, I learned that several conditions could mimic dementia (such as brain tumors, infections, and brain injuries), and convinced everyone that we needed to rule out other possible causes before settling on dementia as a diagnosis.

The scans were ordered. The results came back showing the extensive damage from the stroke that Mom had previously experienced, but there were no tumors. Although the doctor did not feel that the behaviors she was exhibiting were a direct result of her stroke, he felt the stroke could be a contributing factor.

Additional testing was conducted and the results showed that there could be no more denying what was going on with Mom: she was in early-stage dementia. According to the doctor, she had Alzheimer's, the most common form. The word *dementia* is a derivative of a Latin word meaning "apart from the mind," which was so befitting of what was going on with Mom.

According to the Alzheimer's Association's website (alz.org), "Every sixty-five seconds someone in the United States develops this disease." It additionally states that "One in ten people age sixty-five and older has Alzheimer's dementia." Those numbers are staggering and are expected to rise substantially by the year 2050.

It was now confirmed that my mom, Lottie Mae Polk Berry, was part of those statistics. Her diagnosis was based more on the process of elimination—the ruling out of other conditions—than from any one particular test. There was no question as to the validity of the diagnosis, as everything we were seeing seemed to point to dementia. We had to face the fact that the person we had known and had loved for years was no more. We were about to embark on the journey of our lives, and it was not going to be a pleasant one.

According to the Alzheimer's Association, the early stage of dementia is characterized by the following:

- Problems coming up with the right word or name
- Trouble remembering names when introduced to new people
- Challenges performing tasks in social or work settings
- Forgetting material that one has just read
- Losing or misplacing valuable objects
- Increasing trouble with planning or organization

The Alzheimer's Association also recommends that you consult a physician if the following early warning signs of dementia are exhibited:

- Memory loss that disrupts daily life (asking the same question over and over)
- Challenges in planning or solving problems (trouble following recipes or tracking bills)
- Difficulty completing familiar tasks at home, at work, or at leisure (driving to familiar locations, remembering rules of games)
- Confusion with time or place (forget where you are or how you got there)
- Trouble understanding visual images and spatial relationships (difficulty reading or judging distances)
- New problems with words in speaking or writing (struggling with names of once familiar items)
- Misplacing things and losing the ability to retrace steps (accusing others of stealing items)
- Decreased or poor judgment (less attention to grooming)
- Withdrawal from work or social activities (difficulty keeping up with conversations)
- Changes in mood and personality (confusion, fearful, anxious, easily upset)

Lesson: If you or a loved one are exhibiting some of the aforementioned symptoms, a physician may administer a Mini-Mental State Examination (MMSE), which provides a snapshot into whether these behaviors could be dementia. Other cognitive and blood tests, imaging, and neurological exams may also be conducted to rule out other disorders.

Although Mom was initially diagnosed with Alzheimer's, once the Cedar Glen physician learned of her love of beer, the diagnosis was changed to Wernicke-Korsakoff syndrome, which can be caused by a lack of vitamin B$_1$ (thiamine) or chronic alcohol abuse.

Indeed, Mom loved her beer and tended to drink more than she should; however, I didn't feel she drank frequently enough to cause the degree of damage associated with Wernicke-Korsakoff. Admittedly, I am not a clinician and knew that Mom's treatment plan would not be affected by the type of dementia she had, so I didn't make an issue about it. I planned to make an appointment with a neurologist once she was released from Cedar Glen.

Lesson: If dementia is suspected, it is extremely important that you seek a diagnosis from a neurologist who specializes in treating dementia—not someone who just dabbles in it. I can't stress this point enough! By understanding the type of dementia your loved one has, you can see if you are at a higher risk for developing it and learn how to decrease that risk. Also, you can gain a better understanding of how the disease will manifest itself, progress, and obtain strategies for coping with the illness.

Accepting Mom's dementia created a sense of urgency and forced us to act. We knew she would need additional assistance once she returned home, but we didn't know the extent of that need. We decided that, at minimum, someone needed to check in with her during the day while Daniel was at work. Daniel graciously agreed to continue with the evening and overnight check-ins. Thus far, once Mom was in bed, she tended to stay there. We hoped there wouldn't be a need for him to stay with her overnight.

Daniel would ensure her needs were met before she went to bed and again in the morning before he went to work. The rest of us would either call or stop by on our assigned day to ensure that Mom was okay and didn't need anything. Although Nicholas and I still worked (Lewis and Don had retired), we had some flexibility with our jobs and didn't feel we'd have a problem doing our part.

Ravenna was part of my service area for work, so I could check on Mom when I was in town and on weekends. Those who lived closer committed to stopping by to bring lunch or breakfast, or at least check in on her daily. Certainly, if everyone did as he/she committed, Mom would be able to stay in her home for a long time. We were devoted to her while she was at the SNF. Surely, we would be even more devoted to her once she returned home, right?

On one particular day, when I visited Mom at Cedar Glen, the social worker invited me to come into her office. This had not happened before, so I knew it couldn't be good news. She informed me that they take photos of all incoming residents and wanted to show me Mom's picture. The social worker opened a folder, held up the photo, and I burst into hysterical laughter. My eighty-year-old mother was glaring at the photographer as she proudly presented him with her middle finger. It was then that I learned a very valuable lesson.

Lesson: Unapologetically take advantage of any and all opportunities for laughter. They will be few and far between.

When I arrived at Mom's room, she and her roommate Ellen were not present. Looking at the clock, I deduced that they were at lunch. Mom never ventured out of her room alone, so I was sure she had followed Ellen to the cafeteria.

The first-floor corridor of the facility was configured in a square. Once you stepped into the hallway, you could turn left or right and still pass all necessary stops: the nurse's station, therapy room, activity room, cafeteria, front desk, and the offices of various staff members before ending up at your original starting point.

Mom appeared unable to grasp that concept or remember how things were laid out. She could not determine which way to go to reach her desired destination, let alone remember what her destination was. She shadowed Ellen wherever and whenever Ellen left the room.

I decided to go find Mom instead of waiting in the room. As I walked towards the cafeteria, I tried to recall the last time I'd had lunch with her. Embarrassingly, I couldn't remember ever having taken my mom to lunch. That was certainly an "ouch" moment.

When I arrived at the cafeteria, I witnessed something I had not seen before. I stood in the doorway and observed Mom bullying another resident. Mom was making faces and taunting the woman as she talked about her to other residents. I could not believe it.

Initially, I did not intervene because I was in a state of disbelief. How far was she going to take this? I had never seen my mom do anything like this before—although I had heard many rumors of such behavior—and I was greatly concerned. Where was this behavior coming from?

I reached the point where I could no longer be a silent observer. When I called out to Mom, she immediately changed her behavior. She became upset that I had called her out and stated that she had been doing nothing wrong. As we were leaving the cafeteria, per her request, she turned towards the woman she'd been bullying and stuck out her tongue at her. Who was this person, and why was she behaving so poorly?

When I shared the lunchroom happenings with Mom's seventy-year-old cousin, Nina, she told me that Mom had always been somewhat of a hellion and shared stories of Mom picking fights and bullying others as a child. I knew that it was extremely common for persons with dementia to regress, but I didn't expect to begin seeing that regression so quickly. As time went on, more and more of this "unlikeable Lottie" would rear her ugly head.

Mom started to become upset whenever we showed Ellen any attention; if we brought Mom treats, she would become irate if we brought Ellen some, too. Mom also began accusing Ellen of trying to seduce my brothers. This was a very interesting dynamic. On one hand, Mom was upset with Ellen and jealous of her, but on the other hand, she felt dependent upon her.

Cedar Glen just did not have the staff available to give Mom the extra attention she needed, such as getting her from point A to point B when she wanted to go. As a result, she continued to shadow Ellen wherever she went.

Lesson: A skilled nursing facility (SNF) is staffed for rehabilitation. It is not meant to serve as an assisted living or nursing home, providing extra needed services. Staffing is limited.

Within three weeks of being in the SNF, Mom had progressed to the point where she was doing everything for herself. Her motivation to comply with physical therapists was her desire to return home. Physically she was great, although cognitively there was much cause for concern. As she became increasingly agitated at the idea of being away from home, we faced the reality that there was no need for her to remain at Cedar Glen.

She had regained her strength and was walking without assistance. She was performing all of her ADLs (activities of daily living) herself. There was nothing more to be gained if she stayed. Selfishly, we wanted her to stay because we knew she was safe; it bought us time. Of course, Cedar Glen staff encouraged us to keep her there but could not provide a rationale.

Lesson: A facility may want a patient to stay for the full amount of time that Medicare allows and will pay for, regardless of whether the patient really needs it.

I requested and was granted a care conference, which included the director of nursing, the physical therapist, the social worker, and an aide. During the conference, the aide confirmed that Mom was doing everything for herself. She was stronger and just wanted to go home. There was no reason for her to remain at Cedar Glen.

Daniel wasn't excited about the idea of Mom going home. He'd been able to rest better than he had in years, feeling that she was safe and being cared for at Cedar Glen. He did, however, agree that we needed to get her back to where she was happy—unless there was a health or safety-related reason that she shouldn't go home. That meant Mom was going home!

Fear thou not; for I am with thee: be not dismayed; for I am thy God: I will strengthen thee; yea, I will help thee; yea, I will uphold thee with the right hand of my righteousness. Isaiah 41:10

Chapter 7
Going Home

The staff at Cedar Glenn made us aware that as long as Mom was homebound (unable to go anywhere outside of the home due to her condition), she would qualify for in-home assistance. They said a nurse would come by a couple times a week, and Mom would also continue with her rehab services, which she didn't need.

Unfortunately, it was quickly determined that Mom was not truly homebound. Friends came by to take her places, including shopping, church, and out to lunch. Because she was not homebound, the planned supportive services stopped.

It was time to see how well my brothers and I would hold up our ends of the bargain. Would we make sure Mom still got to Mass at her beloved Immaculate Conception Church if her friends were unable to do so? Would we still make regular visits to check in on her? Would we try to keep her life as close to normal as possible? We had the best of intentions, but would we follow through?

Lesson: Self-assess the motives behind the decisions you make. Determine whose best interest is being served. What are you willing to do to maintain or improve the quality of life of your loved one?

In the year before Mom's admittance to the hospital, her driver's license had been surrendered. This was not an easy task, as she had fought us tooth and nail. As mentioned earlier, we had noticed dings and dents on Mom's car regularly, and she could never remember how they occurred.

One day, while going through some of her papers, I noticed a copy of a police report that showed that Mom had struck a pedestrian while turning a corner. She became agitated when I questioned her about it. "I am a grown-ass woman and don't have to answer to you about anything. You just need to mind your own damn business," she said.

Certain I would not get additional information regarding the accident from Mom, I asked some of my contacts to gather more details. Mom had been deemed "not at fault" for this incident, but I learned of another disconcerting scenario. Mom had hit another vehicle while trying to park at a shopping center. She had moved to another spot after hitting the vehicle, shopped, and then returned home. Someone had witnessed the incident, recorded her license number and vehicle information, and contacted the police.

The police went to her home and she was able to convince them that she did not know she had hit the car. When they asked why she had changed parking spots, she said, "I saw a car leaving a spot that was closer to the front door, so I moved." They had accepted her explanation, or had they? This was one of a few times where I wondered if the reputation of my brother John was helping to keep Mom from experiencing the consequences of her actions.

My siblings and I were so concerned about Mom's apparent decline in driving ability that we tried to get her physician to sign paperwork stating she was unable to drive. Mom threatened to fire her if she did, and the doctor took that threat seriously. As more dings and dents occurred, we tried to see what other options were available to assist in our endeavor.

Lesson: Although a physician may agree that your loved one shouldn't be driving, don't expect them to sign the paperwork needed to take the keys away. Their loyalty is to their patient, not to you.

At one point, Daniel had hidden Mom's keys. In retaliation, she called the police, who came to the house and questioned Daniel. Because there was no record of her being impaired and unable to drive, they mandated that Daniel return her keys to her. No one had deemed her incompetent; she still was making her own decisions. We didn't like it, but that's the way things were. It was a conundrum. It was like being held in limbo, just waiting for a tragedy to occur.

As Mom became more confused, we became more concerned. She may not have been bad enough to be deemed incompetent from a medical standpoint, but from our point of view, she was not well enough to make important decisions. The fact that she experienced moments of clarity did not help our case at all. She had the uncanny ability to go from being completely confused to lucid whenever her mental capabilities were being challenged.

It wasn't until Mom's ophthalmologist identified a major problem with her vision (which was becoming increasingly worse), that we were finally able to get the deed done. She had lost her eyeglasses and needed to get a new pair. The ophthalmologist determined it was time for her yearly eye exam, which was conducted prior to her receiving new glasses. During the exam, he discovered that Mom's vision had seriously deteriorated since her previous exam due to macular degeneration. He told her that she absolutely should not be driving as she was now legally blind.

Here is the kicker. Mom said, "If my eyes are really that bad, I guess I can't be driving." This is very important to note. Instead of someone telling her not to drive, she decided that she would no longer drive. The ophthalmologist had told her she *shouldn't* drive, but not that she *couldn't* drive. That made all the difference in the world in terms of surrendering her license. It allowed her to be the decision-maker in a choice that would affect the remainder of her life. She felt she was in control, although she wasn't.

Think about it. For the last several years, there were so many things over which she'd had no control. Heart attacks, strokes, deaths, illnesses, and injuries had become a part of her daily life. She was watching friends and relatives die. She was losing the ability to perform tasks that had once been second nature for her. Loved ones weren't coming by to see her as often because the visits were challenging. She needed to feel like she was in control of something, and the decision to give up her license helped her feel that sense of control. It was only semantics, but it was important to her.

Lesson: The elderly lose so much as they age. It's important for them to feel they have as much control over what happens in their lives as possible. Where they are, you may one day be. Keep that in mind.

Since Mom's divorce, she had become fiercely independent. The loss of her license also meant the loss of independence. She had to depend on someone else to take her anywhere she wanted to go, as opposed to being able to get up and go whenever and wherever she chose. As I look back, that was when we began to see a more significant decline with her. She displayed a deep depression that I had not seen in her before. Although I tried to be empathetic, there was no way I could truly understand the impact that giving up her license had on her.

Once Mom returned from her stint in rehab, we had to step up our game. Initially, we all did a good job of pulling our weight, putting ourselves on a Saturday schedule for taking Mom and Daniel shopping in the morning and Mom to Mass in the afternoon. Nicholas also volunteered to take her to Mass on Monday mornings, with her friend Barbara taking her to breakfast with the girls afterward and then home. So he'd know that Mom had a ride home, he would call Barbara on Sunday evenings to ensure that she would be attending church the following day.

Because I was driving from Richmond Heights, a suburb of Cleveland, I would spend my entire assigned Saturday with Mom. After shopping, I would put her groceries away and take her to lunch before taking her to Mass. These lunches became something I looked forward to because she seemed to enjoy them so much.

Mom's restaurant of choice was the Evergreen Buffet in Kent, Ohio. She was quite the people-watcher, and the array of persons coming to

35

her favorite Chinese buffet always garnered comments from her. However, those comments kept me on edge. You see, whatever filters she had left were beginning to diminish. She would say whatever came to mind, and she didn't care who heard her. She would also stare unabashedly.

When I would ask her not to stare, she would say, "I'm not staring. I'm looking." When I'd ask her to stop talking negatively about people, she would say, "If they didn't want to be talked about, they should have worn clean clothes, brushed their hair, lost weight, etc." The list was endless. I would tell her that I could never take her to my neighborhood to eat out of fear that she'd get us hurt. She'd just laugh and continue with the stares and comments.

It was during those lunches that I connected with Mom in a way we had never been able to before. She began to tell stories of her past, laughing as she'd relay different incidents to me. It was after one of our lunches when she said, "I love you always" for the first time. From that moment on, whenever I'd tell her I loved her or say goodbye, she'd respond with those words, "I love you always." I looked forward to hearing those words. I knew that a time would come when she would not be able to utter them, so I treasured them.

Although I valued my lunches with Mom, it was also during those lunches that the changes occurring with her would become more evident. Mom had always had a challenging personality, but now I was seeing something different. I can't tell you exactly what it was; it was just different. I could tell that Mom was slowly progressing in her dementia journey, and that deeply saddened me. Anticipatory grief—grieving over what was to come—would become a regular part of my existence and I didn't like it. Although I wanted to live for and appreciate today, I couldn't help but think about tomorrow.

I knew that tomorrow was not promised, but I feared what tomorrow would look like. Despite our concerns, my brothers and I still neglected to plan for the future. If we didn't think about it, we didn't have to act upon it.

Take therefore no thought for the morrow: for the morrow shall take thought for the things of itself. Sufficient unto the day is the evil thereof. Matthew 6:34

Chapter 8
More Change

As time passed, many subtle changes would come to light. Mom's short-term memory became worse. The accusations became more frequent. The phone calls and paranoia were increasing. Her depression became greater, and the sadness in her eyes broke my heart.

Mom used to enjoy visiting my home occasionally for a few days every month or two. George and I have a vast backyard that garners a menagerie of wildlife. She would sit in our family room, which has glass doors that extend the width of one wall, for hours looking at and identifying the different animals. She would become excited every time deer ventured into the yard (a common occurrence), commenting, "They probably taste real good!"

Mom became more uncomfortable coming to my home. Initially, I thought it was because she hated climbing the steep steps leading to her bedroom. As a result, we converted our first-floor office to be "her room" whenever she visited. However, that didn't change her thoughts about spending the night at my house. I later came to realize that she didn't want to visit because she was becoming more confused with regards to her surroundings. She was beginning to have difficulty finding her way around my home, which was causing her additional anxiety.

The goal of bringing her to my home, in addition to wanting to spend time with her, was to give Daniel a break. He would be able to rest, knowing Mom was being well cared for and safe. Ironically, she began to use Daniel as an excuse for why she wanted to stay home or go home. She would say, "I've got to go home to keep an eye on Daniel in case he needs something." Once she got that thought in her head, there was no changing her mind.

Because of Mom's growing discomfort at being away from her home, I switched from having her come to my home to spending a night or two at her home at least once per month. Again, my goal was to try to give Daniel a break. I scheduled my overnights when it was my turn to take them shopping and made a sort of ritual of it.

After work on Fridays, I headed to Ravenna for my sleepovers with Mom. Daniel usually ordered from our favorite pizza place, Guido's. Mom would eat, visit for about an hour, and then head to bed. She was going to bed earlier and earlier those days. Once she went to bed, Daniel and I would have an opportunity to talk about what was going on in our lives and the changes we were seeing in Mom.

I would awaken on Saturday and clean out Mom's fridge, ridding it of expired foods and old leftovers. This gave me a snapshot of how Mom had been eating . . . or not. Initially, she was still doing light cooking for herself so there wasn't a great deal of waste. Daniel would prepare a preliminary grocery list consisting of staples, and I would add to it based upon what foods I knew she was eating and the items that I tossed every time I visited.

Mom was a creature of habit, so there were items that we always added to the list: sausage, bacon, eggs, milk, biscuits, Pop-Tarts, cereal, and Miller High Life beer, to name a few. I came to realize that the foods she purchased were her staple foods because they were so easy to prepare. Miller's was a point of contention among the siblings: most did not want to deprive her, and one refused to supply her. If we didn't get it for her, friends would supply it later in the week anyhow. It just wasn't worth the tantrums—yes, literal tantrums—she'd throw if we didn't get it for her.

Next, I would check Mom's lottery tickets for winners. Playing the lottery was a not-so-guilty pleasure of hers, and she had three different three-digit numbers that she always played. No, I'm not going to share those with you because she would be angry if I did!

As time progressed, Mom had a great deal of difficulty determining whether she had winning numbers. I had a designated space where she was to place her lottery tickets, and I would check them before going to the grocery store. I eventually added the Ohio Lottery app to my phone so I could quickly scan the tickets and determine whether they were winners.

I hated that she wasted so much money on the lottery, but she once told me that playing the lottery and drinking beer were the only pleasures she had left in life. That made me so sad. She hadn't gone walking since breaking her ankle. She used to enjoy doing word search puzzles, but her vision failed her and she was no longer able to do them. She used to love putting picture puzzles together but no longer had the mental acuity required to complete them. And now, she could no longer drive.

My poor mom had experienced so much loss that I was not going to make a big deal about her choosing to spend money on lottery tickets. She was not taking food from anyone's mouth or depriving anyone of shelter. Playing the lottery brought her pleasure, which she had little of over the past several years. Although I may have felt it was a waste of money, it was her money to waste.

Lesson: Make this your mantra: "If a behavior is not hurting them, you, or anyone else, don't sweat it."

After the grocery list was completed, the refrigerator cleaned, and the lottery tickets checked, we'd head to the grocery store. She insisted upon walking from the parking lot to the store, stating that she needed to do as much as she could for as long as she could. We'd then get her riding cart and begin our adventure.

First, we had to cash-in/purchase her lottery tickets. Next, we'd venture to the fresh fruits and vegetables. Even though I ended up tossing her spoiled and rotten fruits because she wasn't eating them, each time we shopped she insisted upon buying more. If it looked good, she wanted it. She was very much an impulse shopper.

In the prepared foods section, I would ask Mom to "stay in the lane" as I picked up some of her regular weekly items. She always looked at the fried chicken and soups and said the same thing: "I will come back and get it before we leave, so it will be hot for our lunch." It was rare that we went back to make those purchases because she'd forget about it by the time we reached the checkout. Truth was, either Daniel would buy us lunch, I would take her out to lunch, or I would cook. If she had chosen to purchase hot food, it would have been cold by the time she ate it. If she remembered wanting something specific once we reached the checkout, I'd always go retrieve that item for her. Most times, she wouldn't remember.

Once home, I would put the groceries away and it was time for lunch. Most times we went out, usually to the Evergreen Buffet. Going to a buffet eliminated the frustration of trying to make a selection from a menu. Too many choices on a menu made her anxious; trying to remember what each item was and whether she liked it was frustrating and challenging for her.

Buffets eliminated that anxiety. She could see the food items and get whatever she thought she liked, and if she later found that she didn't like an item, she didn't have to eat it. She always had a mixture of chocolate and vanilla ice creams and Jell-O for dessert.

Going to a buffet went against one of the principle lessons I'd learned about dementia regarding choices, but every rule does not apply to everyone. Buffets worked for Mom.

Lesson: Don't present too many options to a person with dementia. Offer no more than a couple of choices at a time and afford the person ample time to respond. For example, "Would you like an apple or an orange?"

As I mentioned earlier, I had really come to enjoy my lunches with Mom. She was a real character, and I would become tense while waiting to see what would come out of her mouth as she observed other patrons. Despite that, we seemed to connect during those times. I'd show her pictures of my granddaughter, Ann, and discuss what was going on in her life. Mom would reminisce about her past, which seemed more like yesterday than yesteryear as time went on.

She began to confuse Ann with my daughter Lynn, interweaving various components of their lives. She would think Ann lived with me, although she recognized Ann was Lynn's child. She would remember Lynn was married, but constantly reverted to Lynn's time as a child or teen, asking me about her schooling and such. It became more challenging to hold a conversation with Mom. I had to remember to go with the flow

Lesson: Instead of trying to bring persons with dementia into the present, go with them into their world and try to enjoy the journey.

Charity suffereth long, and is kind; charity envieth not; charity vaunteth not itself, is not puffed up, doth not behave itself unseemly, seeketh not her own, is not easily provoked, thinketh no evil; rejoiceth in the truth; Beareth all things, believeth all things, hopeth all things, endureth all things. Charity never faileth. 1 Corinthians 13:14–8a

Chapter 9
Who's Liz?

In 2015, Mom's dementia presented many challenges. I can recall members of my work team using the term "pleasantly confused" when describing some of their hospice patients who had dementia. It didn't take long to see Mom was not going to be pleasantly confused. She was confused, but there was little about her personality that was pleasant. That may be a terrible thing to say, but it's the truth. Based upon my experiences, the persons closest to the one with dementia are the ones who experience the brunt of the anger, confusion, and meanness.

Mom began misplacing numerous items. As more things disappeared, "Liz" appeared. According to Mom, Liz was Daniel's girlfriend and was responsible for anything that went "missing." Mom believed that whenever she left home, Daniel brought Liz over to steal her things. Mom would go to church on a Saturday afternoon, only to come home and cuss Daniel up one side and down the other for letting Liz into her home. She was convinced that Liz existed and was stealing her things at every opportunity.

As it turned out, we eventually discovered that Liz was a real person. Although Mom had worked with Liz years earlier, Daniel had never had any interactions with her. It was a case of Mom taking someone familiar and implanting her into what was confusing and unfamiliar to her. Liz showed up often during the next few years. She was someone who would have a presence until the end.

Mom's accusations of people stealing from her were incessant. It was painful witnessing the exchanges between her and Daniel. The more he denied, the angrier and more accusatory she became.

Lesson: You can't reason with a person who has dementia, and you are not going to win. When you are accused of stealing something, redirect them and offer to help them find the item. You might say, "You know, I saw that the last time I was here. I can't remember where it was but let me help you look for it." If you can't find it, take a long time to look. Chances are, your loved one will have forgotten about it by the time you stop looking. Don't argue. Redirect!

We quickly learned that Mom was hiding things because she was fearful that items were being stolen. Unfortunately, she could not remember that she'd hidden the items and denied having done so. We developed a habit of looking for "missing items" in drawers, shoes, cupboards, and other unlikely places whenever there was an accusation of theft.

Lesson: It is easier to accuse someone of stealing than to admit that you don't know where you placed something.

Side Note: If you have not already done so, now is the time to make sure you have access to all important documents. One suggestion is to make copies and return the copies to the place your loved ones typically keep them; you keep the originals. Also, make sure you have copies of keys and are aware of all accounts, safe deposit boxes, insurance policies, etc.

When I'd observe Daniel becoming upset when Mom verbally assaulted him for one reason or another, I would touch his arm and say, "It's not about you. It's the disease." What I sometimes failed to realize was that I could leave the situation when I became upset, but Daniel couldn't. He lived this all the time, and I was becoming more concerned about what this ordeal was going to do to him. I would tell him that it was useless to argue with Mom. She was living her reality, and no matter what he did or said, she believed that what she was saying was true. Then my husband became her target.

Mom began calling me to say that George was coming to her home and asking for money. The first call went like this:

"Hey," said Mom. "How are you doing?"

"I'm fine. How are you doing?" I asked.

"Is your husband mad at me?" she asked.

"No," I replied. "Why would he be mad at you?"

"Because he came out here asking me for money, and I told him no," she said.

"Mom, George doesn't need your money."

"Maybe he needs money and you don't know about it," she said.

"Mom, I have access to our accounts, and he does not need your money. He did not come out to ask you for money. And if he needed money, he would go to his dad," I said.

"So," said Mom, "Are you calling me a liar?"

"Mom, I am working, and I can't talk right now. I will call you later." Of course, I never called back.

These accusations continued for about a month. I found myself becoming upset each time I got a call, or when I'd visit and the topic came up. Although I knew this was all related to her illness, I couldn't help myself.

Lesson: No matter how personal it seems, it's not personal.

As a creature of habit, Mom did not like anything or anyone interfering with her routine. One of those routines involved going to breakfast with her lady friends after Monday morning Mass. Unfortunately, one day I didn't think of that when I scheduled her a doctor's appointment on a Monday morning. She was livid!

45

Because of my work schedule, and the fact that I wanted to be present for her appointments, I didn't want to change the appointment time. I told her that we would catch up with her friends for breakfast after her appointment. That appeased her, so we went ahead with our plans as scheduled.

True to my word, after her appointment we went to Burger King, where the ladies were meeting that morning. Unfortunately, because her appointment had lasted longer than expected, the ladies had gone by the time we got there. Mom instantly began to pout until I told her that we could still have breakfast together. We went to the counter and she ordered a burger and fries. I interrupted her, telling her that breakfast was still being served and she couldn't have a burger and fries.

The clerk immediately corrected me, saying, "Lottie can have whatever she wants. If she wants a burger and fries, she can have a burger and fries." That moment was when I really recognized the value of Mom living in a small town. People knew her and appeared to genuinely care about her. I helped Mom to her seat and went back to the counter to pick up our order. The clerk wanted to know who I was. I told her I was Lottie's daughter.

She asked why Mom wasn't driving any longer, and I told her it was due to her failing eyesight. She then told me stories of how my mom would drive to Burger King, park way in the back, and not in a particular spot. She also told me that Mom would sometimes come through the drive-through, order, and then drive off without paying for, or retrieving, her order. Although staff were concerned—and most knew two of Mom's sons—they never shared this information with anyone.

As Mom and I were chatting during breakfast, I asked her if she remembered ordering things and driving off without getting what she'd ordered. She laughed and said, "All the time." Surprisingly, she was not only able to answer all my questions, but she answered honestly. I asked if she had ever gotten lost while driving, and she had. She shared that she liked going to Walmart in Kent, but oftentimes couldn't remember how to get home. When I asked what she would do, she said she would ask someone how to get to Central Hospital, which was down the street from her home. She felt if she could get to the hospital, she could get home.

Isn't it amazing that she could remember that her home was down the street from the hospital and had the presence of mind to ask how to get there? She admitted that the reason she was having trouble parking was because she couldn't see the lines. As a result, she just parked far away from the other cars. When I asked if she had shared any of these stories with her friends, she laughed and said, "Yes." As one who was in contact with Mom's friends regularly, I was initially angry that they had not shared that information with me. Then I realized that they'd had no reason to tell me. Mom was their friend; I wasn't.

Lesson: The elderly look out for their own. They are not going to share any perceived negative information about their friends with you.

This breakfast with Mom was quite pleasant and informative. However, I became more concerned about what I did *not* know about what Mom had been experiencing than what I *did* know because of what I'd learned. I thought about her ability to appear competent whenever it was necessary, and how she was able to convince someone of her innocence when she was guilty. I thought back to the parking lot incident, when she had hit a car while parking and moved to another spot, and wondered how she had the presence of mind to tell a story that kept her from being arrested.

Although my concerns were growing, there were also many unexpected blessings during our breakfast together. Mom's anxiety vanished. She was extremely pleasant, talkative, and spoke the truth. I was grateful for it and wondered how many bonding experiences I had missed out on by not spending more time with Mom. Although we hadn't had what I'd call a close relationship, it was respectful.

It was because of this particular breakfast that I decided to make opportunities to take Mom out to eat, and not just on my scheduled Saturdays. These meals would provide us with an opportunity to bond as never before, and Daniel would receive much-needed reprieves . . . if only for a couple of hours.

Lesson: Don't look back on what could or should have been. Live in the moment and enjoy the blessings that unfold.

Honour thy father and mother; which is the first commandment with promise; that it may be well with thee, and thou mayest live long on the earth. Ephesians 6:2–3

Chapter 10
Food for Thought

S oon, the accusations of theft and speaking badly of others brought me to the point of not wanting to be around Mom. As challenging as it was, I'd think about what Daniel was experiencing. If he could deal with her every day, surely I could spend a couple of hours with her. I did not want to become yet one more person who chose to stay away from her because she made me uncomfortable.

Although I knew it was the dementia that caused her to do much of what she did and say much of what she said, it was no less painful. In my heart of hearts, I believed that some of what I was witnessing was inherently inside her. I have no scientific basis for that opinion; it was just a feeling.

Our drives to lunch seemed to be the worst times. To say I was tense during those drives would be a gross understatement. To avoid responding to her rants, I clenched my teeth so tightly at times that my jaw ached for hours. One drive in particular comes to mind.

Per usual, Mom had spent the entire ride talking about how Liz and Daniel were robbing her blind. Then she said that Lewis had begun asking her for money. She said that he had spent all his money on women and was crazy to think she was going to take care of him after that. I wondered if Lewis was going to be her new target and dreaded the thought that soon, things were going to get worse.

When we arrived at the buffet, I parked and walked over to assist Mom in getting out of the car. She quickly told me to let her do it herself stating, "If I don't use it, I'll lose it." She then asked me to walk in front of her, which I thought was odd.

After we were seated and beverage orders were taken, we walked up to the buffet. Again, Mom asked if I could walk in front of her and said she would follow me. Initially, I was trying to get her to go in front of me or alongside me so I could assist her. Then I remembered something.

> **Lesson:** Peripheral vision and depth perception can diminish as dementia progresses.

Mom wanted me to walk in front of her so she could see where she was going. I was her "guide dog," in a sense. As I looked behind me, I could see that she was having some challenges judging distances but didn't want my assistance. It was challenging for me to let her be, but she wanted to do for herself. Then there was lunch.

I knew my mom was a bully, but now I was learning how much she liked to stare. Because she lacked a filter, she commented unfavorably about people as they would go through the buffet line. If they were obese and overfilling their plates, did not appear clean, were scantily dressed, or whatever, Mom had something to say. I shushed her constantly. I would tell her to stop staring and, as was becoming her norm, she'd say, "I am not staring, I'm looking." I often told her that I was fearful she'd get us hurt one day because of her rude comments and stares. She'd respond, "I'll kick their asses!" She'd probably make a valiant attempt at doing just that, I thought.

People at the buffet gave her dirty looks, but no one ever said anything. I wanted to put a sign on her head that said, "Please forgive me. I have dementia and am not responsible for what I do or for what comes out of my mouth."

Once she got over the initial phase of speaking poorly of people, things would take a turn for the better. We would make small talk about anything and just laugh. She had given my granddaughter the nicknames of Little Squirt, Nutty Buddy, and Stinky Butt. I wondered whether those were terms of endearment or names she used when she couldn't remember Ann's name.

She wanted to know everything about Ann and never tired of looking at photos I'd captured of her on my phone. I again noticed how much she was intermingling the lives of Ann and my daughter, Lynn.

In Mom's mind, Ann and Lynn had now morphed into one person. It made for very challenging conversation as I tried to discern whom she was actually speaking of or asking about.

Lesson: Persons with dementia may reach a point where once familiar faces are no longer familiar to them, including their own.

As our lunch progressed, Mom reverted to her original behavior. Her devilish side would come to the forefront. "Oh, look at that fat pig piling that food on her plate. Look at how that slob is dressed. He could have at least combed his hair." The barrage of insults continued throughout the remainder of our time at the restaurant. When I asked her to lower her voice, she said, "You don't tell me what to do!" I'd threaten to leave, but she would assure me that she was not going anywhere.

Why would I continue to take her out in public if her behavior was so troubling? I took her because for the first time in my life, I was feeling close and connected with my mom. When she wasn't being inappropriate, she was wonderful. We had conversations about everything, even though she did not remember the conversations moments later.

It was during those lunches that I felt loved, and I showed love. I was looking at the mom that I didn't remember having while growing up. We were creating a bond. I didn't have many positive memories from my childhood, but we were creating new ones. I began to treasure those lunches.

Chapter 11
Decisions, Decisions, Decisions

In 2016, Mom became obsessed with planning and paying for her funeral. Almost every time she saw me, she would tell me that she wanted to make her funeral arrangements. The idea made me uncomfortable.

I don't know why I reacted that way. As a hospice worker, I saw time and time again the negative impact of poor end-of-life planning, or lack of planning altogether. I saw the strain it placed on families when they had to try to figure out what their loved ones would want or guess what their final wishes would be. It was as if people felt that completing advanced directives and funeral planning would result in their untimely deaths.

I saw firsthand the stress placed upon families when there was disagreement about what to do, or how to do it. My dad had repeatedly said that he wanted to be cremated. He hated the idea of "being eaten by worms" and stated he wanted to be burned, put in a box, and kept on someone's shelf.

Fortunately for me, he had written down his wishes in his own handwriting and had the document notarized. My dad died long before people were routinely talking about living wills and medical powers of attorney. He'd been ahead of his time in many ways. Even though his wishes were clearly stated, there were still persons who tried to challenge the decisions I'd made.

In addition to having the desire to be cremated, Dad requested that there be no funeral. He asked that a small, uplifting memorial service be held instead. Again, this resulted in much contention. My firm response to questions regarding any decisions was, "I am following Dad's wishes. If you have any issues, take them up with him." I then produced his handwritten document to silence anyone questioning what and how things were being done. I was extremely grateful he had made his wishes known.

Knowing the benefits of preplanning, I couldn't understand why I was so hesitant to do what Mom was asking. Perhaps deep down I was exhibiting the same superstitions many others had. Maybe I felt that her death would be hastened if we planned her funeral and burial. I considered myself to be a well-educated, logical woman, but I was not thinking logically at all. I was thinking emotionally, and my emotions were keeping me from honoring my mother's wishes.

Eventually, she stopped mentioning funeral planning and I was grateful for that. If she didn't mention it, I didn't have to think about it. I didn't have to do anything.

During 2016, we saw a continued decline in Mom's cognitive abilities. Her symptoms were intensifying, and she became more confused and combative. Dreams became more vivid, and she was having difficulty distinguishing between what she had dreamed and what was real. I remember a specific instance when she called me, extremely distraught, stating that during the night someone had come and buried a lot of bodies in her backyard. She was scared that the person was coming after her.

After a lengthy conversation, Mom was finally able to recognize that she had been dreaming. Surprisingly, she laughed about the incident, saying, "I was dreaming, wasn't I?" I was thankful she was able to come to that realization on her own. If I had tried to convince her, it would have led to an argument where she would accuse me of trying to make her think she was crazy.

It was also in 2016 that I began to see a major decline in my own health. I was being diagnosed with illnesses I'd never heard of, like Ménière's disease and trigeminal neuralgia, to name a couple. I was fatigued all the time and often felt as if I were going to fall asleep while driving to appointments for my job. I began a list of my symptoms and made an appointment with my primary care physician.

I also began praying even more than I had before. I felt like I was dying, and I was not ready. I told God all the reasons that I felt He should let me live. My husband had survived prostate cancer and we had plans to grow old together. My daughter needed my support with Ann. I wanted to be around to see my stepdaughter, Yvonne, marry and have children. I needed to be there to continue to help my mom. I had so many reasons for asking Him to spare me.

In the interim, George began trying to convince me to retire. Eight years my senior, he had been retired for over ten years and always hated the idea of my going off to work while he stayed home. It didn't bother me in the least. He was an excellent money manager; we didn't suffer one bit financially after he retired. He was also amazing at doing things around the house. I used to tease him and say, "If I'd known you would have been this great of a househusband, you could have always stayed home."

In hindsight, I believe he was becoming concerned about me and my health. I was holding a full-time job, taking care of our home, helping to care for my mom, and providing back-up support for Ann. It may have seemed like a lot, but I didn't mind it at all. I loved my roles as wife, mom, daughter, and nana, and the jobs associated with those titles. However, I knew something was wrong with me and was concerned that my time on this earth was going to be limited.

When I went to my scheduled doctor's appointment, I presented my list of symptoms to the physician. After very briefly looking at the list, she told me to pick the two symptoms that were the most bothersome and to make another appointment to discuss the others. In all honesty, I can't remember what the remainder of our conversation entailed because I had decided, at that moment, that I would not be returning to her and would need to begin searching for a new doctor.

In August, as luck or divine intervention would have it, three of my friends mentioned seeing a functional medicine doctor at the Cleveland Clinic. Each one spoke of how functional medicine doctors were intent on finding the root causes of health problems, as opposed to merely treating symptoms. Each of my friends had raved about their treatment plans, how much their overall health and well-being had improved after seeing these doctors, and how their regimens continued to work wonders for them.

As my own health declined, I called for an appointment with the Functional Medicine Department. As you could probably guess, appointments were being scheduled out months in advance, and there was no availability until November. I took that appointment and prayed for strength as I felt pulled in so many different directions. Because I am not a complainer, no one had any idea of how bad I was feeling. George knew that I was very fatigued and was constantly providing support in that area, but that was all he knew.

He continued to press me to retire, and I continued to give him reasons why I shouldn't. There were things I wanted to buy before retiring, like new living room furniture and carpeting. There were places I still wanted to visit, which he had me list. This amazing man put things in place to allow me to get the things I wanted—and made plans to go to the places I wanted—but I still made excuses. I didn't want to retire because it had taken me far too long to get to a place where I could be independent.

Having been married and divorced by the age of twenty-one, to say that I had struggled as a single mom would be a gross understatement. If not for the financial and emotional support of my parents and strong faith in God, I would not have survived that time. The thought of having to rely on someone else to care for me again made me feel sick to my stomach. I had finally reached the point in my life where I could do for myself if I had to. I could buy what I wanted without thinking twice, go where I wanted, and do what I wanted. Why would I let go of my nice income to have to go on a strict budget?

I began to pray very hard about the idea of retiring. Health insurance was not cheap, and because I was only sixty-two at the time, the idea of paying a large sum of money for health insurance for three years was not at all appealing.

George did some investigating and number crunching until he came up with a financial plan that could work. Still, I resisted. Then, I felt as if I had heard God reminding me of how far he had brought me. I felt Him show me a fast track of the past forty years of my life.

I reflected on the struggles I had experienced and how I overcame them. They formed me into the person I am today, a person I liked and respected, and one that others did, too. If I had not gone through those challenges, I don't feel I would have a heart of compassion or heart of gratitude. I saw that the person I am is because of what I have gone through and God's grace.

Whether through my temporary stint on welfare after the divorce, or through support from my parents, I have always been provided for. I may not have had everything I wanted, but I've had everything I've needed. That was a blessing.

It became clear to me that, of late, I had been living a life of excess. I had more than I needed. If I continued to work, I'd be working for more excess and clutter. It was August 2016 when I decided to retire—a decision that George was happy with. Before I could change my mind, I wrote up a formal letter advising my boss that I would be retiring in February 2017. Giving him that letter made my decision more real. In my mind, there was no turning back.

Behold the fowl of the air: for they sow not, neither do they reap, or gather into barns; yet your heavenly Father feedeth them. Are ye not much better than they? Matthew 6:26

Although the decision was made, I would be lying if I said I was happy about it because I wasn't. I resigned myself to the fact that the career I had worked so hard to establish would soon be over. Despite how I felt internally, the plans for retirement continued and, as luck would have it, my retirement was right on time. Not only was my health declining more, but Mom's dementia was also advancing.

She became even more paranoid about her finances and called me several times daily to inquire about them. She'd say that someone (meaning me) had taken all the money out of her bank account and that she was going to call the police and have that person arrested if her money was not put back immediately.

I would access her account via my computer, review transactions with her, and would share her current balance. I'd then tell her that the next time I was in the area I would take her to the bank where she could obtain a printout of activity. Although I had the capability of printing out the activity myself, she would doubt the validity of what I gave her. Going to the bank and receiving this same information from the banker would alleviate her anxiety.

We began seeing other interesting changes in Mom. She was becoming extremely forgetful, not just with conversations we'd have, but also with whether she'd eaten, bathed, brushed her teeth, etc. She became moody and had a lack of recall. Her personality began to seriously change, and she had difficulty determining the times of day.

Mom began calling her friends at all hours of the night, which was upsetting and bothersome to them. They would tell her not to call them if it was dark outside, but Mom wouldn't recall the conversation.

Although I didn't receive the nighttime calls, Mom began calling me multiple times daily saying that people, specifically Daniel, were stealing her belongings or bringing strangers into her home. The calls always ended with a threat to call the police to have someone arrested. It was challenging to talk her down from these calls, but most times I was successful at redirecting her. If she mentioned an item had been stolen, I would tell her that I had moved it the last time I was in her home and would retrieve it for her the next time I visited.

Some people challenged me by saying that I should not be lying to her, but I disagreed. I was redirecting her and taking away the anxiety that she was experiencing. She rarely remembered the phone conversation, but if she did, I would look for whatever item she thought had been stolen when I visited.

My being less than truthful was hurting no one. In reality, it helped to placate Mom and create a less stressful situation. It was evident that she was now moving into middle-stage dementia which, according to the Alzheimer's Association, is characterized by:

- Forgetfulness of events or about one's own personal history
- Feeling moody or withdrawn, especially in socially or mentally challenging situations
- Being unable to recall their own address or telephone number or the high school or college from which they graduated
- Confusion about where they are or what day it is
- The need for help choosing proper clothing for the season or the occasion
- Trouble controlling bladder and bowels in some individuals
- Changes in sleep patterns, such as sleeping during the day and becoming restless at night
- An increased risk of wandering

With the changes in Mom's behavior, I realized it was time to honor her wish to plan for her funeral. I couldn't bring it up because she would view it as my thinking she was going to die and that I was trying to take her money. Instead, I had to wait for the next time she brought up the idea and be ready to act accordingly.

Ironically enough, during this extremely challenging time I had my November appointment with the Functional Medicine Department of the Cleveland Clinic. After extensive testing and a complete medical history, it was discovered that I had late-stage Lyme disease. In addition, I tested positive for multiple coinfections transmitted by ticks.

To my surprise, my Functional Medicine physician referred me to an independent physician who specialized in the treatment of Lyme disease and other tick-borne illnesses. Because this specialist was the only one in the state of Ohio, I was unable to get an appointment until the following April. I wasn't concerned about the delay in treatment, as it was determined I had been living with this disease for many years. Waiting another few months was no big deal. In the interim, due to my compromised immune system, I was placed on a variety of supplements to assist with fatigue and other issues.

Chapter 12
The Mysteries of the Mind

Although officially diagnosed with dementia in 2008, there was a dramatic decline in Mom's mental health in late 2016 and 2017. Her short-term memory became worse. The repeat questions were incessant, and the frequent calls were unnerving. She continued to have vivid dreams, with the one involving the bodies being buried in her yard occurring multiple times.

During one episode of discussing this with me, she became so distraught that I had to go to her home. However, when I reached her, she didn't even remember having had a conversation with me. After I had been with her for a while, she looked at me and asked, "Am I going crazy? Something is wrong with me, but I don't know what it is. My mind just is not right." I tried to explain that she had dementia and help her understand what that meant, but I believe she was more confused after my explanation than she was before it. Eventually, I would just tell her that she had an illness that affected her brain and caused confusion. That explanation would appease her until she'd ask again.

Mom had reached a point where she was no longer able to rationalize anything and had a great deal of difficulty comprehending most things. She was frustrated and, I think, afraid. It was so sad to witness. She knew that she was slipping away but couldn't understand why, or how. I told her that this may have been a long-term aftereffect of her stroke, believing that it would be easier for her to understand than dementia.

Lesson: I believe that persons with dementia, understand at some point that they are slipping away but don't have the capacity to understand why. Imagine how distressing that must be!

In April, I had the first appointment (of what would be many) with my Lyme Literate Medical Doctor (LLMD). We met for a few hours as he reviewed pages of my medical tests and medical history, telling me that I'd had more positive test results for tick-borne illnesses than he had ever seen. Because George and I traveled quite a bit, I could not tell the doctor definitively where I contracted the illness, but I was able to recall when the telltale bull's-eye rash had appeared on my calf.

Based on the information I provided, my test results, and my medical history, he thought I'd had the illness for more than fifteen years. He stated that the treatment would be lengthy and couldn't guarantee a cure. He felt that we would be able to keep symptoms at bay and was hopeful that I would eventually become Lyme-free. Only time would tell.

Lesson: There is a tremendous amount of controversy surrounding Lyme disease and how to treat it. Much of this was made clear to me by watching the movie *Under Our Skin.*

On May 25, Mom had an appointment scheduled with her neurologist. It was non-eventful, as was always the case of late, but the conversation was unusual.

"Lottie, can you tell me what day it is?" asked the neurologist.

"Hell, I don't know," said Mom.

"Who is the president?" he asked.

"Kennedy," she replied.

He continued. "If the person in front of you dropped a twenty-dollar bill, what would you do?"

"Keep it!" she said.

"What year is this?" he asked.

"1928," she replied.

I chuckled as I couldn't understand why these questions were being asked. We had already established that she had dementia, so her answers were always going to be wrong or inappropriate. If nothing else, the sessions would cause her to laugh. I never quite understood why, but they did.

After her doctor appointments, I would take Mom to have blood work drawn and then to breakfast at Megan's Family Restaurant, which was one of the places she frequented with her friends. The staff not only knew her by name, but they also knew what she ordered regularly. No menu was needed, which was great. Mom would get her regular meal of crisp bacon, eggs over medium (not runny but not hard), hash browns, lightly buttered toast, and a cup of coffee.

Mom would always complain that the eggs were over or undercooked, the bacon was too crisp, and no matter how little butter they put on her toast, she'd scrape it off while complaining that it was too much. Even though she complained, she ate most of it and asked for a container to take the remainder home.

While much was the same with this breakfast, it was also different. Out of the blue, she said, "I want to pay for my funeral. I don't want you all to have to pay for it, and I want it to be the way I want it." Her funeral home of choice, Shorts-Spicer-Crislip, was close to Megan's, so I let Mom know that we would go pay for her funeral as soon as we finished eating our breakfast.

Fortunately, we were able to speak with a representative and my mom was lucid. She knew she didn't want to spend a great amount of money on her funeral and told the representative not to show her anything expensive. A devout Catholic, she knew her service would be held at the Immaculate Conception Church and needed to be officiated by the son of her late godmother.

Mom selected a beautiful pink casket with a blue floral inlay and received a bill of $9,377.18, which covered all funeral and burial expenses. Her bank was one block away from the funeral home, so we immediately went there, obtained a cashier's check for the full amount of the funeral expenses, and returned to the funeral home to make the payment. I had the representative make five copies of all paperwork to ensure that I and each of my siblings had a copy. It was important to me to give my brothers copies of not only the funeral expenses, but also any large monetary transactions. I did not want anyone questioning what was being done with Mom's money.

When Mom expressed a desire to purchase her funeral flowers as well, I wouldn't allow it. I let her know that was something her family would want to do for her. She didn't argue. She then stated that she wanted to purchase her headstone. I told her that she would not be able to do so at that particular time, but I reassured her that I would schedule an appointment to purchase the headstone soon.

I was amazed that Mom was able to stay "with it" and focused throughout the entire funeral planning. Unfortunately, by the time we returned to her home, she couldn't remember anything that had taken place in the hours before, asking when her appointment was and if we could go to breakfast. I assured her that we had already seen her doctor and presented her with the leftovers from Megan's. She ate just a few bites before announcing that she was full.

I placed copies of all transactions in envelopes for each of my brothers and put them in the location where we placed all important information we needed to share. I called each of them to let them know what had taken place earlier that morning. After I was assured Mom would be okay, I returned home (I'd retired as planned in February).

Although Mom was the one with the desire to make her own arrangements, I was the one who was feeling relief. I was grateful that my brothers and I would not have to go through the ordeal of deciding what to do and how to do it when that time came. Now, as was the case with my father, we had our road map. Our only task would be to adhere to the plan Mom had laid out. I had no doubt that we would do just that.

After a while, Mom began calling every morning to ask whether certain things had occurred or if she had dreamed them. It was amazing to witness how her mind appeared to be working—or not. Was she actually being rational? How was it possible to be so confused one moment and reasonable the next? There was no rhyme or reason. It just was!

Lesson: Don't try to make sense of the seemingly senseless.

I later learned, after one of my overnights with her, that she enjoyed watching Court TV and murder mysteries while in bed. Oftentimes, she fell asleep with the television on, which I believe fed into her subconscious. As a result, I suggested that Daniel turn off the television once she fell asleep. I didn't hear any more about her backyard cemetery after that.

During the previous several years, we had consulted with a few neurologists who claimed to specialize in dementia. The visits were fairly brief, but the MMSE was administered at each visit regardless of whom we were seeing. They would also ask a series of questions and have her try to conquer certain tasks. The neurologist would ask, "Lottie, could you please draw a clock face for me? Who is the president? What year is this?"

Mom typically ran out of patience after the third or fourth question or task saying, "Why are you asking me all of these damn questions? Are you stupid or something?" While I initially didn't understand why they kept administering the MMSE since she always failed it, I later learned it was one tool used to determine how the disease was progressing.

It was interesting to me that, although her answers were never correct, there were certain questions that she consistently answered the same way. Kennedy was always the president and the year was 1928, the year of her birth. The neurologists would recommend various medications like Namenda and Aricept for symptom control (anxiety, depression, confusion, etc.), which we would try. Unfortunately for her, the side effects seemed to be worse than the symptoms. She experienced more confusion and muscle cramping, became more agitated, developed insomnia, and a host of other side effects that caused Daniel to make the decision, with my blessings, to discontinue the medications.

Lesson: It's a good idea to keep a medical/symptom journal. Note the behaviors/symptoms you are seeing, the time of day you are seeing them and what, if anything, happened before the behavior/symptom you saw. Take this information with you to physician visits.

As Mom began having more difficulty keeping her medications straight and taking them on time, Daniel began to manage them. Before going to work, he prepared containers of meds, which he'd label and place at the table where Mom ate breakfast. I would call Mom later in the morning to make sure she had taken her medications and ask her to read to me what the label said.

Daniel administered late day/bedtime medications when he returned home from work. This system worked well for all involved for quite a while . . . until it didn't.

Lesson: Sometimes, difficulties experienced by the elderly are because they are not taking their medications or are not taking them properly. Put a system in place to ensure your loved ones are getting what they need when they need it.

I will lift up mine eyes unto the hills, from whence cometh my help. My help cometh from the Lord, which made heaven and earth. Psalms 121:1–2

Mom didn't speak of her funeral arrangements for months after she had made them until something jarred her memory. On August 18, Mom called and told me that my brother Lewis was going to have bypass surgery and asked if I could take her to the hospital. She didn't have any details regarding dates, times, etc., but she was sure the surgery was going to take place in a couple of days. When I asked her how she knew about the surgery, she couldn't remember who told her, but she knew she had been told by someone.

My initial thought was that she'd probably had another dream that seemed real to her, but I decided to investigate to ensure that was the case. It was not uncommon for folks in my family to have surgery and not tell anyone about it until after the fact. There was a very real possibility that Mom was correct in what she was saying. I sent Lewis a text advising him what Mom had said, and he confirmed that he indeed was scheduled to have surgery on Monday, August 21 at Union Hospital in Cleveland.

When I asked if it would be okay for me to bring Mom to the hospital, he said it was, but on the condition that I not become involved in his care. He did not want me to hear anything that the doctor said regarding outcomes, stating he wanted the doctor to speak only with his son, Anthony. That was a difficult promise for me to make because I am the inquisitive one, the one who does research, asks questions, and questions decisions. He made it clear that I was to do none of those things, and I agreed to honor that request. People tend to be secretive about their medical conditions and may choose not to share that information with anyone other than those who need to know. I had to respect his choice.

I decided to get Mom the day before the surgery because it was scheduled for early in the morning and, if she were at my home, she would be able to sleep longer. Because of her difficulty with stairs, a bed was set up in the downstairs office. I knew that if she woke up during the night she would be confused and disoriented, so I decided to sleep on the living room couch that was adjacent to the office area.

As I predicted, Mom awoke multiple times during the night and had no idea where she was. I had left a trail of lights so she could find her way to and from the restroom, but that didn't help at all. She would awaken, get out of bed, and just stand in the doorway until she heard me call out to her. I had to remind her who I was, where she was, and accompany her to and from the restroom. At one point, I heard quite a bit of commotion coming from her room. When I went in, she was standing at the back end of the office and appeared to be very confused. When I asked what she was doing, she replied that she was looking for the bathroom. I was so glad I walked in before she sat down in my chair!

As you might guess, I got no sleep that night. I was concerned about my brother and afraid that Mom would somehow manage to get out of the house. I let her sleep as long as possible before waking her to go to the hospital. I helped her dress, fixed her breakfast, and had her make a bathroom stop before we headed on our way.

We arrived at the hospital and checked in at the sign-in desk to see if Lewis (who was riding with his son Anthony, granddaughter Margo, and Daniel) had arrived yet. The receptionist checked her list and said that Lewis's surgery had been canceled. My first thought was that they had notified him and that he neglected to call me, but I quickly learned that was not the case. The receptionist asked me to call Lewis to tell him that his surgery had been canceled, but I refused. I told her that Lewis would have questions that I would not be equipped to answer and that he was probably close to the hospital already. I was a little miffed that he had not already been notified of the change but managed to hold my tongue. This was not my battle to fight.

When Lewis arrived, I didn't let him know what I had been told. Instead, I watched quietly as he walked to the desk and was told by the receptionist that his surgery had been postponed. Lewis had no idea what was going on and made a series of phone calls. Within fifteen minutes after his last call, he received a call back advising him that his surgery would go on as previously scheduled. He never volunteered any details, and I didn't ask.

Anthony, Margo, Daniel, Mom, and I sat in the waiting area as Lewis was taken back to prep for surgery. We laughed and spoke about anything but the surgery as we waited to see him before he would be taken to the operating room. Everyone wished him well as he was taken down for surgery.

It took approximately four hours for the surgeon to come out and inform us that the surgery had been successfully completed. As I had promised Lewis, I stepped away as the surgeon shared details of the surgery. This was very challenging for me, and I wondered whether Daniel had been given the same instructions I had but had chosen to ignore them. I had a mile-long list of questions but knew that I needed to respect Lewis' privacy. He needed to be the one to make decisions about what information he wanted to share and to whom he wanted to share it.

When I returned to the room after the surgeon left, Anthony told me that the surgery had gone well, but the surgeon had cleared seven blockages as opposed to the quintuple bypass we had initially been told about. I was unaware that there were seven arteries within the heart, so I wanted to question what was being said. Instead, remembering my promise, I held my tongue. The important thing was that Lewis had successfully come through the surgery and appeared to be doing well.

I had brought Mom's things to the hospital with me so that I could drive her and Daniel home without having to stop back at my house. I was sure Anthony and Margo would want to stay at the hospital longer than Daniel and Mom would want to. After Lewis was out of recovery, we said our goodbyes and headed to Ravenna. I silently thanked God for yet another victory.

Daily updates from Anthony assured me that Lewis was doing well . . . until he wasn't. Early on the morning of August 24, the house phone rang. Instinctively, I knew this was not going to be a good call. Daniel, who began with his usual "Sis," was calling to let me know that Lewis had died earlier that morning and that everyone was on their way to the hospital. Damn him! I began to sob and asked how Mom had handled the news. He said that she had handled it better than he had expected and told me that Don would be bringing them to the hospital.

George tried to comfort me as I hung up the phone, but I couldn't be comforted. It seemed so unfair. My dear mother would have to bury another son. All I could think about was how close she had been to Lewis. Although she always complained that he lied to her or allegedly kept asking her for money, her eyes still lit up when he entered a room. I would remind her that Lewis was retired from his own company and that he was a city councilman. "He doesn't need your money," I would tell her. I knew not to argue with her, but for some reason, I always got upset when she claimed people were asking for her money. Now all I could think about was how she would handle the loss and what impact it would have on the progression of her dementia.

My siblings and I, along with Anthony, our niece Margo and Don's sons Richard, Thomas, and Lucas, met in Lewis' room. His body had not yet been taken, so we were all able to say our preliminary goodbyes. Everyone began sharing their favorite Lewis stories as tears were shed. Even though we could see he was dead, I think we were still somewhat in denial.

The hospital staff were great, allowing us to spend as much time with Lewis as we needed. They had also set up another room for us to meet in, so after about an hour, we moved to the secondary room. Mom was fairly quiet, and Anthony just seemed to be lost. I believe he was in shock. I began to wonder, What if his surgery had been postponed as the hospital had originally advised us? Would we still be here under these circumstances or would we be visiting a Lewis who was on the mend?

I don't know why we hung out at the hospital for so long. It was as if we were waiting for something else to happen, but what it was, I don't know. Anthony seemed to be at a loss for what to do next. Recognizing that Anthony was Lewis' closest relative, I knew funeral planning was going to fall upon him. When I asked him what I could do to help, he replied that he had no idea what to do. I asked if he wanted assistance with funeral arrangements. Relief flooded his face and he thanked me with a hug.

The next day I met with Anthony and Mom to discuss the arrangements. Anthony let me take the lead, again saying that he had no idea what to do. He was grateful for the input Mom and I provided.

Mom was surprisingly lucid during this planning process. You may ask why we involved her at all. Mom was the one with the local connections. We were not aware of Lewis' actively attending any church, and Anthony confirmed that Lewis was not affiliated with a church as well. Anthony also said that he could find no important papers such as a will, last wishes, insurance, etc. Therefore, he would have to rely on Mom to use her church and, possibly, for financial support. A switch seemed to go off in Mom's head, enabling her to think clearly. We decided on the preliminary dates of the calling hours and funeral and finalized a time to go to the funeral home to make the arrangements.

When we met at the funeral home, we selected a casket and made plans for the arrangements with the funeral director. Anthony learned that as a city councilman, Lewis was entitled to a small life insurance policy, which the funeral director felt would cover the cost of the funeral. Mom made it clear that she would take care of any excess expenses, including the cost of the repast. Anthony, who had no idea what a repast was (a meal served to the family and friends of the deceased individual after the funeral), expressed his gratitude for the support.

I instructed Anthony that we needed to meet with the church pastor to discuss the service. As with the service for my brother John, Mom wanted the son of her godparents, Deacon Tom Peters, to officiate the service. We scheduled our appointment to meet with Reverend Pierce, Pastor, and Deacon Tom the following day. I decided to stay overnight with Mom instead of traveling home. It was during this meeting that signs of Mom's dementia reappeared.

When Mom saw Reverend Pierce, she told him that she hadn't seen him since their plane ride. Although he was aware that Mom had dementia, he responded, "We've not been on a plane together." She then reminded him that they had sat next to each other when they were coming back to Cleveland from Mississippi, to which he responded, "I have never been to Mississippi, and I have never been on a plane with you."

Even as I was silently mouthing, "Remember, she has dementia," Reverend Pierce continued to debate the issue of the plane ride with Mom. The more she told her story, the more he refuted it. I finally could stand no more and just took control of the conversation, reminding everyone that we were there to plan a funeral service. After about half an hour, our task was completed. We had selected readings, assigned roles, and finalized all plans. I was left with the task of preparing the obituary (per Anthony's request) and the program for the service.

Reverend Pierce offered to allow us to have the repast at the church hall, but because it held only seventy-five people (tightly), we would be holding it at the Ravenna Elks Lodge. Lewis had been a member and Anthony had already secured permission for the repast to be held there.

The funeral was scheduled for September 2, with calling hours scheduled for the night before at the funeral home. Next, Mom and I went to Guido's to order the food for the repast. After selecting the menu, paying, and making delivery arrangements, we had lunch and returned to Mom's house. I sent a text to Anthony advising him of the status of everything and reminding him to review the obituary I had prepared and make whatever changes he deemed necessary.

Once I was confident that Mom was doing well, I returned to my home exhausted and hoping that Anthony would complete his assignment. I hated being last minute and was anxious to have the obituary completed and copied. I also needed to make arrangements for someone to serve the food. Unfortunately, Guido's had multiple bookings for the day of the service and even though they had no problem preparing the food, no servers were available.

Normally, I would have been able to count on my best friend, Lena, to handle this for us, but she would be leaving soon for her son's destination wedding. George and I had been scheduled to attend but, obviously, we had to change our plans. Amid my planning, I received a call from my friend Donna who offered to handle the serving of the food. God's timing is perfect!

Donna and I discussed the details and arranged a time for her to go to the Elks Lodge to meet the caterer, and I let her know that I would be dropping off tablecloths around that same time. I contacted Anthony to advise him that everything was set for the repast. He had approved my draft of the obituary, so the only thing left to do was to add it to the program and have copies made.

I was amazed at how well Mom had been doing up to this point. She occasionally asked, "Whose funeral are we going to, Lewis' or Butch's?" Butch was John's nickname. "I know it's one of them," she said, "But I can't remember which one." I gently reminded her that we would be attending Lewis' funeral and that John had died years before, to which she responded, "That's right."

I would oftentimes catch Mom speaking to Lewis. She would say, "I sure do miss you son. I really miss your smile and your laugh." I was becoming anxious because I was waiting for the release. She had not yet shown her emotions, and I felt they may be lurking just beneath the surface. Because of her dementia, I had no idea how those emotions would manifest themselves or what impact this experience would have on her.

I spent the day of the wake with Mom. Knowing she would be stressed about getting ready, I wanted to be there to assist her. New outfits and accessories had been purchased for Mom for the wake and the funeral. She bathed (sometimes a challenging feat when dealing with someone who has dementia), combed her hair, and ate something before I helped her get dressed.

Lesson: Sometimes, persons with dementia become attached to certain articles of clothing making it difficult to have them change clothes. It's a good idea to purchase multiples of items you notice are their favorites. This might make changing clothes an easier task.

Fortunately, she liked her new outfit and was satisfied with the way she looked, since I hadn't allotted any time for foraging through her clothing for an alternative choice. I reaffirmed that she looked good, and we waited for my husband and Daniel to come to the house so we could head to the funeral home. Once they arrived, we headed on our way.

Anthony, Leigh (one of Lewis' daughters), Margo, Nicholas, Meg (Nicholas' girlfriend), and Don arrived right on time. We all walked into the funeral home together for our first viewing of Lewis. Mom touched him and told him that she loved him—and was still very composed. I was confused as I led her to her seat. Anthony looked as if he were still in shock and just going through the motions. He asked me what he was supposed to do.

I had forgotten that this would be Anthony's first time in the lead role at a wake and funeral. I explained that at the appropriate time, people would be coming in to greet the family and offer condolences. I let him know that as the person closest to Lewis, people would want to be sure they could meet him and speak to him. As such, he needed to be in the parlor, unless he felt he needed a break.

He asked where he should stand, and I told him wherever was comfortable for him. I reminded him that we were all there to support each other and that we would be able to get through this together. Mom just sat quietly, taking it all in . . . or not.

I was standing near the casket looking at the flowers as people began to filter into the room. Of course, everyone shared their stories about Lewis as they walked by and offered their condolences. My brothers and I gave each other sideways glances when we were told things that were difficult to believe, oftentimes choking back laughter. We knew the real Lewis.

The biggest moment of the night came when my mom yelled across the room, "LaBena, get out of the way. You are holding up the line." Mom, who seemed to be enjoying the attention she was receiving, managed to make me feel about an inch tall by uttering only twelve words. I was extremely embarrassed; however, her comments lightened the mood. Everyone but me seemed to get a nice chuckle out of it.

When my brother John died, we were at his wake for hours after the scheduled time because of the hundreds of people who came to show their support. He had touched many people through his work. For this reason, Anthony decided to schedule two wakes: one from 2:00 to 4:00 p.m. and the other from 6:00 to 8:00 p.m. Because Lewis was a city councilman, Anthony felt that many people might show up, and the two viewings would avoid the same issue we'd had at John's wake.

There had been a steady stream of people during the first wake, but it was not overwhelming in any way. Because of the break in between, the family was able to head back to Mom's for a bite to eat before the second viewing time. Surprisingly, everyone was in good spirits, including Mom. This time with family seemed to be good for all of us, even though we were tired and somewhat dreading the requirement to sit through another two hours at the funeral home.

The pace of the second viewing was extremely slow with fewer than twenty people coming to pay their respects. There were several times when family members were the only ones present. It was during those times that we began to tell stories. Everyone had a Lewis story, some more favorable and funny than others. These stories resulted in laughter that I sometimes found disrespectful until I thought about it. During those moments, his life (the good, bad, and ugly) was being celebrated.

Mom sometimes interjected her own story, which would catch us off guard and make us smile because we were unsure what was fact and what was fiction. At eight o'clock, we said our goodbyes, planning to meet at the funeral home for one final family farewell to Lewis in the morning before heading to the church. Mom walked to the casket, kissed Lewis, and said, "See you tomorrow, son."

I again planned to stay the night with Mom so that I could ensure she'd have the help she needed before the funeral. She ate a little before heading to bed, not showing much emotion. I wondered if the lack of emotion was due to her dementia. Was she not remembering from one moment to the next that Lewis had died? Did she not understand what death meant? Did she not know how to show what she was feeling?

Mom was already awake when I got up on the morning of the funeral. She said that she had washed up and was hungry, so I fixed her breakfast and coffee. I got cleaned up and dressed while she ate, helping her do the same after I'd finished. Like the day before, we waited for Daniel and George to arrive so we could go to the funeral home for the final family viewing. We were all unusually quiet on the drive, and I reminisced about this same drive when John had died.

We waited in the parking lot until everyone had arrived before going into the funeral home. We all gathered around the casket and took turns giving Lewis a final touch, kiss, or word before heading over to the church for the service.

The service went smoothly until it was time for us to leave for the cemetery. As I was walking with Mom and holding onto her arms, it was as if her legs had suddenly disappeared from underneath her. George had gone to retrieve the car, so Mom wouldn't have to walk too far, and my siblings were acting as pallbearers. Thankfully, my father-in-law Benjamin and sister-in-law Marie were nearby to help me catch Mom before she hit the floor. It was as if Mom had just realized that Lewis was gone. She began to sob uncontrollably and cried out for her son. My heart was breaking and I, too, sobbed while trying to comfort her as I led her to a seat with help from my in-laws. I was sure that experience was going to have a very negative impact on her.

When we arrived at the repast after going to the cemetery, Mom had a great deal of difficulty recognizing people. Persons that she had known two days prior were now strangers to her. She asked former sisters-in-law, whom she had known since childhood, who they were. Each time one would cross her path, she would say, "Who are you? Did you know my son?"

She also did not recognize any of her grandchildren. Most had stopped visiting her years earlier because she had been so difficult to be around, but she also didn't recognize those who visited somewhat regularly. She confused Ann with Lynn, and Yvonne with Lena. It was surreal seeing her in this state.

I knew in those moments that our lives were about to take a severe turn. Were we ready?

Peace I leave with you, my peace I give unto you: not as the world giveth, give I unto you. Let not your heart be troubled, neither let it be afraid. John 14:27

Chapter 13
The More Things Change

In early January 2018, Daniel called to let me know that Mom had wandered over to the neighbor's home. Mind you, her neighbor, Mrs. Murphy, had been dead for a few years and her home had been vacant for quite some time. The home was up for sale and fortunately, this happened to be a day where Mrs. Murphy's grandson, Jason, came by to check on it.

This was one blessing in disguise. Another was that even though this occurred in January, it was a fairly warm winter's day. Mom had gone outside, for a reason she was unable to explain, and locked herself out of her home. She was walking towards Mrs. Murphy's house, fell, and was unable to get up. Jason pulled into the driveway, saw Mom and helped her up, and asked what she was doing outside with no coat. With Mom's help, Jason called Daniel to come get her. She had actually remembered Daniel's number!

Mom had initially requested that Jason just break into her house, being "with it" enough that she didn't want her children to know she had locked herself out. Of course, Jason refused and put Mom inside his car while he called Daniel. Since Daniel was working and could not leave immediately, Daniel called Don who hurried over to let Mom into her home. Don then stayed with her for a few hours until he felt comfortable that she would not go out again.

You may be asking why she was home alone in the first place, and I could offer many reasons. Mom was content being home alone and, historically, wandering had not been a concern. My siblings and I took turns calling her throughout the day to check in on her. Now retired, I would take her to lunch and visit at least once per week, as did her friends Barbara and Eunice (who took her to breakfast to meet with some of her former coworkers). She had microwave-ready meals and finger foods at her disposal and a Life Alert button in case she fell. She was content to stay in, bird-watching from her dining room window as she watched the television positioned near the window.

Mom's wandering was a change that was a call for action. I offered to have her come stay with me after I retired. Thankfully—yes, thankfully—she refused to leave her home. The truth was, my mom's behavior had become so challenging that I am sure I would have had to choose between her and George if she resided with us. Also, she was not kind to George, so I felt that I could not ask him to take this on. She wanted to be in her Ravenna home, near her friends. She wanted to be where things were familiar, and I understood that. Whew!

We had a plan in place for when we reached this stage in the progression of Mom's dementia. Our nephew Thomas, who was on disability after a debilitating car accident, agreed to be her sitter during the days . . . for a nominal fee. Daniel would be with her in the evenings after work and during the night. All we had to do was make a call to put the plan into action, right? Wrong. Thomas was not reachable. His number had changed, and we had used all our resources to find him. Although this was going on for only a few days, we didn't feel we could afford to wait for a response from him. It was time to move to plan B. Unfortunately, we didn't have a plan B.

Lesson: Always have a plan A, B, C, D, and E and be ready to put each plan into place at a moment's notice.

We had to look for someone else to begin sitting with Mom during the day. We knew she would be resistant to the idea but felt she couldn't have a choice in the matter if she wanted to stay in her home.

Nicholas, who worked as a human resources manager at a nursing home, began to look at their home care agency as an option. Daniel was going to check with the social workers at Central Hospital for their input. I made calls to friends and former referral sources of mine to secure recommendations, and Don was going to check with his friends and family for suggestions as well. We knew we needed to have someone regularly checking in on Mom or spending time with her. Mom would not like the idea one bit, but we would deal with that when the time came. Oh, yeah. The time had already come!

During our search, we learned how expensive home care was. The lowest quote we received was $16 per hour and the highest quote was $22 per hour. So that's a minimum of $640 per week ($33,280 per year) to a maximum of $880 per week ($45,760 per year). I wanted to show the yearly cost because the progression of most dementias is long and slow. It is an expensive illness in terms of caregiving. Even if we had considered an assisted living or nursing home, we would not have been able to afford it.

Lesson: There is no crystal ball that can predict how long the disease progression will last, when someone is going to need additional care/assistance, or how long that assistance will be needed. Each person is different.

I was now retired and on a fixed income. The same was true for Don. Neither Daniel nor Nicholas were making the kind of money that would enable them to take on a major additional expense. Mom had some savings, but it would be gone in a year at the maximum care rate. We were stressed thinking about what to do. In the interim, we continued to call Mom throughout the day and make periodic physical check-ins.

As it turned out, we found our caregiver in the most unlikely place: Facebook. During the time we were searching, a Facebook friend of mine was soliciting assistance in finding help for her dad, who was declining in health. A few people mentioned the name Meisha and highly recommended her. When I saw her last name, Mars, I realized that I knew her. She was the half-sister of my best friend, Lena. When I called Lena to confirm Meisha's identity, she told me she was who I thought she was and that she had been a professional caregiver for more than twenty years. Lena highly recommended Meisha to care for my mom. Knowing Lena as I do, I knew she would not recommend Meisha, relative or not, unless she was confident Meisha would do a good job.

Normally, I would not have considered hiring the relative of a friend because I would want to avoid any potential conflict that might negatively impact our relationship. However, we were desperate. I contacted my brothers who, like me, were happy with the potential but concerned about how Mom would react. We agreed to tell Mom that she had to accept the support or she wouldn't be able to stay in her home; this was an entirely different conversation which I will get into later. With the approval of my brothers, I set out to see if Meisha could help us. I left a message at the number Lena had provided and awaited a response.

Meisha returned my call and I proceeded to tell her about my mom. I let her know that Mom had dementia and had had her first instance (I thought) of wandering. "Mom is not one of those nice persons with dementia," I said. "She is argumentative and at times very mean. She accuses people of stealing and of having boyfriends, girlfriends, or husbands who steal from her and constantly ask for money. She loves Miller High Life and will do anything to get it. She also loves chicken wings and the Evergreen Chinese Buffet." I realized that I had been rattling off all this information without giving Meisha a chance to respond.

Meisha didn't seem to flinch as I imparted all of this to her. Instead, she related her experiences in dealing with persons with dementia. She seemed kind, patient, and caring. She seemed perfect for the job.

I explained to Meisha that I felt it would be best to start slowly and be with Mom a couple of hours a day for a few days a week. This way, Mom might be open to Meisha perhaps taking her to lunch (or somewhere else) to establish a rapport with her. I hoped that Mom would like her and get used to her coming around. My goal was that by the time Mom's needs increased, Meisha would have established a good relationship with her, and Mom would have developed the level of trust that would enable Meisha to care for her on a full-time basis when needed.

As you could probably guess, a person with Meisha's credentials and reputation had a full schedule. Ideally, I wanted her to go to Mom's home on Thursday and/or Friday mornings. Her friends were already coming by on Tuesdays to take her to breakfast, and I had established a routine of coming by on Wednesdays. As it turned out, Meisha was only available on Monday afternoons. We had to start somewhere, so Monday afternoons it was.

Meisha and I decided it would be a good idea to introduce her to Mom prior to stopping by to sit with her. We planned to do this on the upcoming Saturday so I could be present. It was my turn to take Mom and Daniel shopping, and Meisha would be available to stop by later in the day.

Because the weather wasn't the greatest, I cooked lunch for Mom at her home as opposed to taking her out to lunch on Saturday. I made two of her favorite dishes, chili and fried green tomatoes, in an attempt to butter her up for the meeting. Initially, I was going to discuss the plan while we were enjoying lunch, but decided I'd better wait until closer to the time Meisha was due to arrive. This would result in less sulking and more time to enjoy each other's company.

While we were eating lunch, my stepdaughter Yvonne stopped by for a visit. She had not seen Mom over the holidays and came by to bring Mom her Christmas gift. At first, Mom and Yvonne were having a great conversation and Mom seemed very aware of who Yvonne was. Then, shortly after Yvonne's arrival, Mom began calling her Lena, which was very disturbing to both Yvonne and to me. Yvonne visited Mom regularly, so it was somewhat alarming when Mom didn't know who she was. Yvonne said, "Grandma, you know who I am. It's me, Yvonne." Mom said, "Of course I know who you are, Lena." Yvonne was visibly shaken by that.

As I think back to all I've previously learned about dementia, I realize that this was yet another sign that Mom was progressing in her illness. During so many of my community presentations, family members of persons with dementia shared the pain they felt when their loved ones no longer recognized them. For me, the idea of my mom not knowing me was the thing I dreaded the most about her illness. My heart would break for them, because of what they were experiencing, as well as for me, knowing I would one day feel the same way they felt.

Not knowing me and my brothers was the manifestation of dementia that most concerned me. My feelings of anticipatory grief intensified, but I only allowed myself to stay in that place for a little while. I knew that if I stayed there for too long, I would not be able to see the blessings that could appear along the way. I must admit that I did fight back a tear as I observed Mom in the moment.

After Yvonne left, I didn't bring up to Mom the fact that she hadn't known who Yvonne was. It would have served no useful purpose and would have probably resulted in frustration on Mom's part. Instead, I told her I needed to discuss something with her: that I had a friend who was going to be stopping by occasionally during the week to visit with her. But before I could get another word out, Mom started fussing. "I don't need anyone to come check on me, and I don't want anyone in my house. They just want to see what I have. I'm not a child. You all are trying to get me out of my house, and I'm not having it. I should have never told you about going next door. It only happened once and now you are punishing me for it. This is my house. You need to mind your own business." The tirade went on for a good half hour, with her saying the same things repeatedly.

In the midst of her yelling, Daniel came over and tried to provide some comfort and reassurance to Mom, but she wasn't having it. I then put my foot down and told her this was what we needed to do to keep her in her home. I told her that if she ended up at Mrs. Murphy's house again, they could let the police know that she was not safe being alone. She could be taken from her home. Also, we, her children, could be charged with neglect for recognizing she needed help and not providing it.

I told Mom that we needed to show that we were doing things to ensure her safety at home. I tried to reason with her, although I knew it was a near-impossible task. Experience had taught me the things I was supposed to do concerning dealing with a person with dementia, but I tended to act/react based on what my heart was feeling and not what I thought I knew.

Lesson: You can't teach your heart how to feel.

It's important to note that Mom, like many others with dementia, continued to have moments of clarity. One moment she could be completely confused, only to make perfect sense in the next moment. Such is one of the many mysteries of this illness.

Meisha finally arrived and as I went to let her in, I told Mom to be nice. I am still amazed by what I witnessed next. Meisha worked magic as she spoke with Mom, and Mom was very pleasant and kind to her. She smiled, laughed, and asked Meisha questions. As Meisha was leaving, she asked Mom if it would be ok for her to come back and visit with her, and Mom told her she would love it if she came back.

Meisha and I finalized the plan for her to return on Monday. She would not be performing any duties; instead, she would just try to establish a rapport with Mom. Meisha informed me that she would call me once she got to Mom's so I could have Mom let her in. When Mom had visitors, she used the garage door opener to let them in so she wouldn't have to climb the stairs.

When I returned to the living room, Mom picked up where she had left off earlier. She was convinced we were trying to get her out of her house. She wanted to see her attorney and get us out of her business. She said, "That woman was very nice, but I don't want her back in my house." She also let us know that she was going to get married. When I asked who she planned to marry, she said, "I don't know. It's going to be a marriage of convenience so you all can't tell me what to do." Where did that come from?

I told her that if she got married, she'd have to answer to her husband. She said, "No, I won't!" and continued her tirade. She told Daniel and me that we were horrible children who just wanted to take and take. She insisted that all we wanted to do was get her out of her house so Daniel could move Liz in. She said some very hurtful and hateful things, and I couldn't take anymore.

For the past several months, Mom's response after I'd tell her I loved her was, "I love you always." That night she just glared at me when I said, "I love you, Mom." I was grateful that I could leave when she upset me. Daniel had the unfortunate task of staying with her until she calmed down. I felt sorry for Daniel, but I couldn't wait to get out of that house!

Lesson: It may hurt, but it's not personal.

On Monday, Meisha called my cell as planned to say that she was on her way to Mom's house. Once she arrived, I had her remain on the line as I called Mom to make her aware that Meisha was there for a visit and instruct her to open the garage door. She let Meisha into the house and couldn't have been sweeter. I listened on as Meisha asked Mom if she could take her to lunch. Mom's response was, "Sure. Let me comb my hair first. I didn't know you were coming." I had Meisha hang up Mom's phone and told her I would anxiously await her report after her visit. I also let her know that Daniel had left her fee, as well as lunch money for Mom, on top of the washing machine located in the garage. We didn't want Mom to know Meisha was being paid to spend time with her because she would have been livid.

Mom had become even more anxious about her money, fearing she would outlive her funds. It did not matter what we did to try to reassure her that she would be fine. She would be insulted and upset to know we were paying someone to keep company with her. We hadn't presented

Meisha to her as a caregiver, but as a friend who would be visiting with her. For now, we felt that was the best course of action.

Meisha called me after lunch, as Mom was putting her jacket away, and told me what great company Mom had been. She had a very good appetite and had been extremely pleasant and talkative. Meisha called me again once she'd reached her car to let me know that Mom was resting comfortably in her recliner when she left.

Later, I called Mom to see how she reacted to the visit. Mom said, "Your friend came to see me. She was very nice, but I don't need her to come back. She just wanted to see what I have." When I asked her how her lunch was, she said they had not gone to lunch. Considering that she can't remember lunches with me moments after she's eaten, this was no surprise. I just laughed. She again told me that she appreciated Meisha's coming by (shocker) but reiterated that she need not return. Baby steps!

That evening, when Daniel arrived home from work, Mom ranted and raved about how I had brought his girlfriend into her home. She was absolutely appalled that I could have done such a thing, and thought Daniel and I were working together to get Liz to push her out so she could move in. It was not Mom's habit to speak negatively of me to Daniel, but he sure got an earful that night.

Mom was now confusing Liz with Meisha. To have the nerve to bring this person to her home, while she was there, was to her the ultimate betrayal. Daniel would be hearing about this for a long time.

Meisha continued her weekly visits for the next few weeks, with Mom resisting when I'd call to tell her Meisha was coming. Ultimately, she accepted the visits and seemingly enjoyed the lunches. I enjoyed Meisha's reports about the antics Mom pulled while they were out. Once, she told me that Mom had confronted a pretty young lady who was overweight. Mom said, "You are such a beautiful girl. Why did you let yourself go?" In true Lottie form, she did not hold her tongue. Whatever came into her mind exited her mouth. Meisha said it never bothered her because whatever Mom was saying was true, and that other people just didn't have the nerve to speak so truthfully.

Soon it was again my turn to take Mom and Daniel grocery shopping. The day was non-eventful as we went through our usual ritual. I decided to take a different route to the store this day because I needed to get gas. Unfortunately, it was not a good decision. Mom became anxious and asked where I was taking her. When I responded we were going to the grocery store but that I needed to get gas first, she said I was going the wrong way. "Are you trying to take me to a home?" she asked. I tried to explain that I was going to get gas first, but eventually turned around and went to the grocery store "the right way." Thankfully, I didn't run out of gas and she was happy that her routine was not being altered. It didn't seem like a big deal but, obviously, it was.

Lesson: Persons with dementia value the familiar. Try not to deviate from their routine, as this may result in undue stress and anxiety.

Once we arrived at the grocery store and Mom had her riding cart, we proceeded to the lottery line as usual. We then headed to the fresh fruits where she wanted to buy everything she saw. We followed a very specific order: apples, oranges, grapes, strawberries, and bananas. I could not deviate in any way from that order or she would become confused and agitated.

I reminded her which fruits she still had at home, but I don't know why I bothered. Sometimes she became argumentative, wanting what she wanted, so I would just let her put whatever it was into her cart. I would then have the checkout clerk set the item aside. Mom wouldn't know the difference unless she caught me talking to the clerk. Then all hell would break loose.

Next, Mom went down the aisle containing the prepared hot foods as I grabbed whatever vegetable she wanted. This time, as with all others, she said, "I'll come back before we leave because I want the food to be hot." We didn't go back!

Mom had a unique style of driving her cart. She would move forward while looking sideways. This was a disaster waiting to happen, and we had many disasters. I recall a time when there was a display of bottled beers, six to a carton, stacked neatly atop each other. I happened to look up just in time to see Mom heading towards the display, eyes fixated on something off to the side. I knew I couldn't reach her in time, so I yelled, "Mom, watch where you are going!" You guessed it. Down came the display. Fortunately, no bottles were broken, but beer suds were rapidly seeping from underneath the countless bottle caps.

I rushed over and began to rebuild the display before any of the store staff saw what had happened, scolding Mom for not watching where she was driving. She quickly let me know, "This is not the first time I've knocked something over, and it won't be the last. They shouldn't have put the damn beer in my way. They know I don't have a license." I couldn't help but burst out laughing as I repositioned the last carton of beer neatly in its assigned spot.

Lesson: Don't yell at someone with dementia. It will serve no useful purpose and will just upset them.

Although grocery shopping with Mom was stressful, I always tried to exercise patience. I know that these trips to the store were freeing for her because she didn't get out much. She would wander through the store as if she were strolling through the park, examining anything in her path. She didn't know—or care—whether she needed something. She wanted what she wanted and fought tooth and nail if you challenged her. It didn't matter that she had four rolls of Bob Evans sausage in the fridge or that you had thrown two away because they had expired. She wanted sausage, and you'd better not get in the way of her putting it in her cart.

Because of the challenges Mom was having with cooking these days, she was doing less and less. She would put items in the toaster or microwave and forget to get them once they finished heating. She had even forgotten to turn the stove off a couple of times, but luckily, nothing was on the burner when she had done this. Once, she had also left something in the oven far too long, and Daniel entered the house to find it full of smoke.

As a result, Daniel began to prepare her breakfasts before going to work and dinners after work. She needed only snack items and microwavable meals for lunch. However, anyone looking into her shopping cart would not believe this was the case. When she shopped, she focused on things that she wanted in the moment as opposed to what she was able to prepare.

As she strolled down the meat aisle, I would ask her not to put anything in the cart until she showed me so I could let her know whether or not it was something she already had at home. She'd throw a roast into her cart that no one was going to cook, and while she reached for a six-pack of T-bone steaks, I would put the roast back. As she'd grab a twelve-pack of whole wings, I'd put the steaks back. It was a never-ending cycle. I knew she was never going to cook the items she placed in the cart, and I hated seeing food go to waste. I let her keep whatever I would be cooking for her on that particular day, but I knew almost anything else would end up expired and tossed.

Going down the aisle, I pitied anyone who stopped in her path. Mom did not grasp the concept of right-of-way; she barreled straight ahead. If I asked her to wait or go around someone, she'd say, "They better move." She would oftentimes shout, "You better get out of my way because I don't have a license," laughing as she uttered the words. Although most people found it funny, some did not, and the glares were sharper than any knife I'd ever felt.

As Mom roamed through the prepared foods section of the store, I would rush to secure her nonperishable items. For some reason, she never ventured into those aisles. When I placed those items into her cart, she'd say, "What's that? That's not for me. Who is that for? Why are you putting that shit in my cart?" I'd show her that the items were on her list, and she'd insist she didn't need or want whatever it was. I learned to ignore her but was bothered when I received "that look" from others. You know, the look that says I'm trying to take advantage of my elderly Mom by having her buy my groceries. Shame on me!

Lesson: Don't concern yourself with what people think of you and how you are caring for or dealing with your loved one. They have not walked in your shoes, and most have no clue what you are going through.

The highlight of that particular trip, as with others, was when we'd reach the checkout counter and mom's inner sailor came out. Whatever the balance due would be, it would elicit a profane response from Mom. "Who put all that shit in my cart? I know this isn't all my stuff. Damn it! I'm not paying for Daniel's food so he can feed that damn Liz. What the hell is this shit?" When I'd ask her to watch her language because children were around, she'd say, "I am not saying any more than what they hear at home." She would then continue with her tirade.

Although the cashiers would be entertained, I would be embarrassed. I wondered if they thought Mom really was paying for my groceries. She always gave the impression that someone other than herself was benefiting from the items in her cart.

Lesson: You are going to be embarrassed. Get used to it, and don't sweat the small stuff. There will be enough big stuff for you to be concerned about along this journey.

As usual, we took the groceries home and I put them away. I asked Mom whether she wanted to go out to lunch or have me cook for her. Because she couldn't make up her mind, I decided to make a pot of chili and fry some green tomatoes for her. She had become such a creature of habit that I was sure she'd enjoy what I prepared. She ate hungrily and exclaimed that everything was good. She was extremely grateful and appeared tired afterward. Looking at her, it was hard to believe she was the same woman who had made such a spectacle of herself just a couple hours earlier.

Mom was not as talkative as she usually was. She said it was because she was tired, and she looked tired. I didn't attempt to make conversation with her as I normally did. I was tired as well, so I ate with her, cleaned up, and placed the leftover chili in the fridge. It would make for great lunches during the week. But for some reason, Mom rarely ate leftovers. While cleaning her fridge, I'd often find carryout and other containers filled with what was probably very good food. Part of me wondered whether she was having challenges recalling how to reheat the food or was forgetting the food was in the fridge. I knew she would not admit to it if she was having trouble, so I'd just have to keep wondering. After all, I knew Daniel was providing her with at least two good meals a day.

As I prepared to leave, Mom asked me to call to let her know when I arrived home. She always asked me to do this, but I never did because I knew she napped after lunch and didn't want to disturb her. She wouldn't remember asking me to call anyhow. Daniel followed me down to the garage and thanked me for shopping, cooking, and cleaning up afterward. I always felt his thanks were unnecessary, considering all he was doing for Mom. His thoughtfulness warmed my heart.

At about 9:30 p.m. my phone rang. The caller ID said the call was from Mom. It was unusual for her to call me that late as she always went to bed early. I answered, thinking she had awakened and was calling to see if I'd made it home safely. She sometimes did that. Instead, I heard an unfamiliar voice saying, "Is this LaBena Fleming?" I said nothing, confused by the call. I then heard the voice say, "This is Officer Somebody." I don't recall his name because I was too busy trying to figure out why he was on my mom's phone. He then said, "Don't worry.

Your Mom is fine." I breathed, without realizing I had been holding my breath.

The officer went on to say that my mom had called 9-1-1 and said that Daniel had taken off with his girlfriend; she needed him and couldn't find him. *Officer Somebody* let me know that since Mom had called the police, they were required to do a wellness check. When they arrived, she could not remember calling them and didn't understand why they were there. *Officer Somebody* then asked if Mom stayed alone. I told him she did but that my brother Daniel lived next door and checked in on her frequently and prepared her meals. The officer stated that they had tried to reach Daniel, but his phone was disconnected. I asked him to hold the line as I attempted to call Daniel from my cell. Daniel answered, so I told him that the police were at Mom's house and asked him to go over and call me after the officers left. I then provided the officer with Daniel's correct phone number and let him know Daniel was on his way over. Then the interrogation began.

During the course of his questioning, he said, "Your mom thinks Kennedy is president." "Mom has dementia. It's not uncommon for her to not know who the president is," I said. He asked more questions about her living arrangements as I again explained Daniel's role in her everyday life. When Daniel arrived at Mom's house, the officer ended the call stating he would call me later if he had additional questions.

Why was I feeling so guilty? Perhaps it was the accusatory tone with which the officer spoke to me. I know he was doing his job, but I resented being made to feel as if we were neglecting Mom. I probably should have been grateful for his concern. Maybe next time, and I felt sure that there would be a next time, I would feel more gratitude.

Daniel called later to share what he had experienced. The officers had interviewed Daniel and Mom. They also did a background check on Daniel to make sure there were no reported incidents of abuse. He was extremely embarrassed and angry. I was able to calm him down, reminding him that Mom initiated the call more than likely due to a dream. I reiterated my mantra: "It's the disease, not the person."

Mom responded to the whole situation in an unexpected manner. She thought we had called the police to assist us in getting her out of her home. I was always amazed by the workings of her mind. The thought that something she had initiated had now turned into a conspiracy on our part was very off-putting. This theme would be repeated many times in the coming months. She alerted her friends regarding what we were "trying to do to her," as if she were calling in the troops. She even called her beloved Dr. Kincaid, who had been her neurologist from the time of her stroke until he moved to another city, to tell him of what we were doing and to garner his support.

Upon learning what she was telling people, I again went to the "What will they think?" space. When would I get over that? When Mom was lucid, she was very lucid. She was convincing to listen to if you didn't know her history. Then again, those who really knew my mom knew the person we were dealing with. They knew she experienced delusions and was paranoid. They knew she lacked reasoning skills and was confused. The people who mattered knew our truth, and we had to get to the space where we didn't concern ourselves with those who didn't.

Lesson: Focus on what you know to be true, not on what others think they know.

The Lord is merciful and gracious, slow to anger, and plenteous in mercy. Psalms 103:8

Chapter 14
Here We Go Again

A few weeks after the police incident, there was another occurrence. George and I were returning from church when I realized I had forgotten to turn my phone on. The moment I turned it on, it rang. It was Daniel. He had received a call from Mom's monitoring service the night before telling him that she had fallen. When he went to check on her, he found her on the floor and unable to stand to her feet. He had last checked on her approximately one half hour prior to when she said she was going to bed. She generally slept through the night, so he was surprised to see that she had gotten up.

He helped her go to the restroom and got her back into bed. Sensing things were not quite right, he decided to spend the night on Mom's sofa in case she needed further assistance during the night. Not long after he had fallen asleep, he awakened to see Mom bracing herself in the doorway of her bedroom. She was unable to move her legs and had been incontinent. Daniel decided that something was seriously wrong and called an ambulance to take her to the hospital.

As I'd done so many times before, I said I was on my way. He tried to convince me to wait until he knew more, but that wasn't happening. When I arrived, Mom was resting, and Daniel was sitting quietly. He told me the hospital had ruled out the flu, and they were doing further testing to try to determine exactly what was going on. He said Mom was confused and did not know where she was; however, she was fairly calm. They had done X-rays and a CT scan, as well as taken blood and urine, and he was just awaiting the results.

As I observed all the monitoring devices, I couldn't help but notice how high her blood pressure was. Daniel told me that stabilizing her blood pressure had been a struggle since she'd arrived at the hospital. They had medicated her twice for high blood pressure, but the medications were ineffective thus far. I was concerned that she'd either had a stroke or would have a stroke. I watched her oxygen saturation (O_2) as it registered on the bedside monitoring device. The nurse said that the normal saturation range was between ninety-five and one hundred percent. Understanding that cells needed oxygen to live, I couldn't help but notice Mom's level hovering at ninety percent.

A nurse entered the room and administered another blood pressure medication. Mom's blood pressure was registering at 180/120, which terrified me. This was now the third different blood pressure medication they had administered, but none were effective. Please don't stroke out, my mind screamed as I uttered the words, "When should we be concerned about the O_2 saturation rates?" She replied that as long as Mom's remained above ninety, no intervention was required. She said they wanted it higher, but above ninety was acceptable for someone Mom's age.

As if on cue, it dropped to eighty-nine, and then to eighty-eight. Mom was placed on oxygen. The nurse stated she had been hesitant to do so because it's difficult to wean elderly patients off oxygen once they are on it. She was concerned about the risk for hypoxia, a condition where not enough oxygen is reaching the cells. She educated me on the fact that this could result in organ damage in a short period of time. Placing Mom on oxygen would prevent that from happening.

We had been keeping Don and Nicholas informed about Mom's condition throughout the day and told them that we still had not received any answers. We also let them know that there was no need to come to the hospital; Mom was out of it and there was nothing they could do. We assured them we would make them aware if anything changed.

Several hours later, we had not been made aware of any test results, and they were still unsure of why Mom had been unable to walk. Mom's blood pressure finally began to decrease, and the attending physician decided to admit her. Shortly thereafter, she was moved from the emergency room to a regular room.

Daniel and I stayed with her until she was resting well, and we had made sure everyone knew she had dementia. For some reason, this fact was not being relayed to the various people who were tending to her needs. Go figure! We let the staff know that she would be confused when she awakened and would probably view them as strangers in her home. We considered staying overnight, but the nurse was confident that Mom would sleep through the night due to the medications she had been given. She then assured us that they would be watching her very closely and that we didn't need to worry.

Once we felt that Mom would be cared for properly, we decided to go back to her house. The ride back allowed us some time to discuss the next steps. We knew Mom would not be able to return to her home for a while, so we needed to decide where she would go for rehabilitative services. We had been down this road before, although this time it was different. This seemed so much worse than before.

Daniel was going to solicit input from the social workers at the hospital regarding potential placement. We needed to take the time to see what was available and to look at reviews and ratings. We hoped that Mom was not seriously ill and would be admitted for a minimum of three nights so that Medicare would pay for her stay at whatever rehab facility she went to.

I spent the night at Mom's house because I was hoping to see whatever doctor would be following her while she was in the hospital. The next morning, as luck would have it, I arrived just moments before the doctor came to her room. He was patient and kind, letting me know that Mom had a raging urinary tract infection (UTI), which are a huge deal for the elderly. He said they would keep her there for a few days to ensure everything was controlled before sending her to rehab. Up to that point, Mom had been behaving well. Even though she was sometimes confused regarding her whereabouts, she was neither combative nor argumentative. We attributed that to the fact that she was so ill she just didn't have the strength to fight.

I relayed the updates to Don and Nicholas, and then to Daniel when he stopped by the room on his morning break. During the day, social workers gave him a list of SNFs near the hospital which accepted

Medicare. We spent the evening researching them and making a final decision. Daniel had Mom's power of attorney and had the final say, but he was receptive to suggestions and desired consensus among the siblings.

There were still only two facilities in Ravenna that accepted Medicare: Cedar Glen and Meadow Lands. Meadow Lands' ratings were horrible for both staffing and care, while Cedar Glen received above-average scores in all areas that counted and exceptional ratings in others. Of course, we chose Cedar Glen.

Upon visiting Mom the following day, we noticed she wasn't using her right hand like she usually does. We brought that to the physician's attention, and he ordered an X-ray. She had an ulnar fracture. We couldn't determine when it had occurred, but having had one myself, I knew that most ulnar fractures require no action. Such was the case with Mom. However, they wrapped her wrist with an ACE bandage, which seemed to make her more comfortable.

The physician continued to focus on getting—and keeping—Mom's blood pressure under control and taming the UTI. Although Mom wanted to go home, she was aware that she was not well.

Lesson: When dealing with people who are caring for your loved ones, remember that kindness goes a very long way.

And we know that all things work together for good to them that love God, to them who are the called according to his purpose. Romans 8:28

Chapter 15
Rehab: Round Two

After three full days in the hospital, Mom was released to Cedar Glen. As before, Mom was upset that she had to go to rehab. Although still unable to walk, she insisted she was able to take care of herself at home. This was an emotionally draining experience for all of us. We knew that where Mom needed to be was not where she wanted to be. We also knew there was absolutely no way she could go home.

Mom had a steady stream of visitors those first few days at Cedar Glen. She also had a roommate, which concerned me. I remembered Mom's prior stay in rehab when she thought she was at home and that strangers were breaking in. This time, because of safety concerns, we had requested a private room but were told there wasn't one available. I would later learn that Cedar Glen reserved private rooms for persons who either had infectious diseases or were under hospice care. Even after a nurse had walked into Mom's room and found her sitting on her roommate's bed telling her to get out of her house, she still was not moved to a private room. When the nurse shared that event with me, I let her know that they would be responsible if either Mom or her roommate were harmed as a result of Mom's confusion.

Mom had gone to Cedar Glen on a Wednesday. On Saturday, I received a text from my friend Lena asking if Mom had gone home. I thought the text was odd and suspected that Lena had gone to the facility and found Mom's room empty, although I didn't know that for sure.

Before responding to the text, I called Cedar Glen. The nurse who answered the phone was extremely anxious as she told me she had just called Daniel to inform him that she'd found Mom unresponsive and that they'd had her transported to the hospital. When I asked what she meant by unresponsive, she told me Mom had been staring at the ceiling, was not speaking, and could not squeeze the nurse's hand when instructed to do so.

I packed an overnight bag, kissed George goodbye, and headed to Ravenna. While I was in the car, I received a call from Daniel, reiterating what the nurse had already told me. When I told him I was on my way, he didn't tell me not to come . . . as had been his norm. This made me extremely anxious. This time, I knew, would be different from all the others. I thanked God for giving me a husband who was so supportive and asked Him to wrap His arms around my mom.

I arrived at the hospital and stopped at the information desk, where I was told I needed to don a mask, gloves, and gown to enter the area where my mom was. This was new! As I entered the holding area, Daniel let me know that Mom had been diagnosed with VRE (vancomycin-resistant enterococci), a highly contagious infection that is resistant to many antibiotics. I was told that VRE bacteria live in our intestines and on our skin and that it usually does not cause a problem or require treatment unless someone becomes ill or weak. Mom was both.

In addition to VRE, Mom had pneumonia and her kidney function was compromised. They were also checking her for *C. diff* (Clostridioides difficile), a highly contagious bacteria that can cause swelling and irritation of the large intestine or colon and explosive, foul-smelling diarrhea. We were told it would take a while for those results to come in.

Lesson: Unfortunately, the very places that we go to for care can be the same ones that result in illness.

We wondered whether Mom's issues were the result of her prior stay in the hospital or her brief time in rehab. Fingers were being pointed in both directions, and there was no way of knowing for sure where she had contracted the illnesses.

I glanced at Mom and wondered whether she was strong enough to overcome this, whatever this was. She looked frail and didn't respond when I spoke to her. Instead, she remained in a fetal position with her eyes closed. However, she did manage to offer some profanity anytime anyone moved her for any reason. "Leave me the hell alone, dammit," she would say. Also, she would cry out in pain when she was moved.

Previously, Mom had fallen multiple times while in the hospital and in rehab. She would forget that she couldn't walk and try to stand. In Mom's case, restraints could not be used. As stated on Medicare.gov, Medicare prohibits the use of restraints "unless they are used to treat your medical condition." And because Mom moved quickly, her attempts to stand would often result in her ending up on the floor quicker than anyone could reach her. We suspected she may have injured herself in one of her falls and that may have been why she cried out when moved. Mom's incontinence had also worsened while in rehab, and I wondered if that was due to the UTI or if it was an indicator that her dementia was progressing.

It was close to 3:00 p.m. when I arrived at the emergency room (ER), and Daniel had been there with Mom since 2:00. We didn't speak much. I think we were both going over so many scenarios in our mind that we were just trying to process everything. Suddenly, a physician appeared in the room. Although he introduced himself, I don't recall his name. He went over the many things that were confirmed to be wrong with Mom and questioned her code status. Cedar Glen had said that Mom was a full-code patient, meaning that they were to do everything possible to keep her alive/revive her, including CPR. He then proceeded to let us know what was involved in CPR, saying, "Her ribs will be broken."

I was more than familiar with the various code statuses because I had taught them as part of my job with HWR. I was having flashbacks to the number of times I had said, "CPR is not like what you see on television where someone presses on a chest for a few moments, breathes a couple of breaths, and the patient is good as new. There is oftentimes physical damage done to the person as a result of the CPR, including broken ribs. CPR is a violent act. Besides, depending upon how long it takes to revive a person, that person may not be left whole physically or mentally." Without even realizing it, I was reciting those words aloud to Daniel.

The doctor wanted us to rethink Mom's code status. He looked serious, and I thought of how difficult his job must be. At one point, I told him he was making me feel as if he didn't think Mom was going to get better. He said he wouldn't be surprised if she got better, but that she could get much worse before she got better. I wondered what "much worse" would look like. She looked like she was at death's door already. I didn't want to see "much worse." He told us he would give us some time to process what we'd been told. He then left the room saying he would return shortly.

As Mom's health care power of attorney (HCPOA), this was Daniel's call. What a horrible position to be in! He wanted to do what was best for Mom, but also honor her wishes. Mom's wishes changed frequently. One moment she'd say that she wanted the doctors to do everything to save her, and the next moment she'd say that she didn't want them to restart her heart if it stopped. Daniel and I agreed that Mom's quality of life had diminished to the point that we didn't feel she would want to be revived if her heart stopped.

When the doctor returned, Daniel told him to go ahead and make Mom a DNRCC-Arrest (Do Not Resuscitate, Comfort Care-Arrest). That meant that although we didn't want them to do anything to hasten her death, we did not want her heart restarted if it stopped beating. We wanted her to be kept comfortable and to be allowed to die naturally. I let Daniel know that on more than one occasion, Mom had said she did not want her heart restarted if it stopped and didn't want a machine keeping her alive. I think that information made him feel better.

A little later he asked if I thought he'd made the right decision. I assured him that I agreed with him one hundred percent. Mom hated being in the hospital and in rehab. She'd be devastated if she were confined to a nursing home. We would just have to continue to pray for direction and guidance.

At about 11:00 p.m., another physician entered the holding area and told us that Mom was being moved. He said it was a step down from the intensive care unit, but that she'd be in a room right outside of the nurse's station that would enable her to be closely monitored. Mom, at this point, still had not opened her eyes but continued to deliver profanity to the nurses who were providing care. We had been keeping Don and Nicholas updated with each new piece of pertinent info and advising them not to come to the hospital.

Once Mom was nestled into her new room, Daniel and I decided to leave for the night and planned to return in the morning. We didn't speak much in the car. I think we were both wondering if this was going to be the last trip to the hospital. We should have known better, because Lottie Mae Polk Berry was not only a badass, she was a fighter. She had set a goal of living to see her ninetieth birthday, and that's just what she intended to do.

I had felt for months that my mom was not long for this world. I questioned whether those feelings were God's way of speaking to me, or whether I was just speaking to myself. I doubted that she would make it to ninety. I'd had that same feeling before she became ill. Still, I wondered if what I was feeling was God preparing me for what was to come or whether it was just me thinking about what was, or was not, to be.

When we arrived at the hospital on Sunday, not only was Mom sitting up in bed, but she was also feeding herself. I had previously expressed concern over what I perceived to be vision changes and her limited use of her right hand. It bothered me to see that Mom was wearing as much food as she had probably eaten, but she was eating. She was also angry. She just wanted to go home. If we heard it once, we heard it a thousand times, and each time was just as painful as the first.

A physical therapist came to work with her while we were there. Mom could barely swing her legs over the side of the bed and as she tried to stand, her legs just wobbled and trembled. It was obvious that she could still bear no weight. I reflected on how the physical therapist at Cedar Glen had told me that Mom had taken fifteen steps utilizing a walker, and I wondered about the validity of that statement. I couldn't imagine that she had gotten so much weaker in such a short time, but then I remembered what she was battling. *C. diff* had now been confirmed, so she was riddled with infection. She was a fragile, eighty-nine-year-old woman who had pneumonia, VRE, a UTI, and *C. diff.* Of course, that would cause extreme weakness and an inability to walk.

After the session, during which she'd verbally abused the therapist, she was exhausted. Daniel and I told her to just go to sleep. After about five minutes, she said, "I told you I was sleepy. Get the hell out of here!" So, we left. Walking down the hallway, we crossed paths with Nicholas. We shared all updates and let him know Mom was sleepy and told us to "Get the hell out of here." He chose to visit anyhow, later advising me how guilty Mom had made him feel. She had told him that, after everything she had done for us, she couldn't believe what we were doing to her. It made him feel horrible. Me too!

Later, when I was sharing my feelings of guilt with Lena, she reminded me that it was our job to make the decisions that Mom was not capable of making herself, regardless of how we felt. We knew she would not be safe at home, even with help. Since our primary responsibility was to keep her safe, we needed to keep her where she was for now. We knew she would be returning home if she became stronger. That was everyone's goal.

In the midst of all this, Daniel and I agreed that Mom would probably need full-time care if and when she returned home. I reached out to Meisha to see if she could recommend a full-time caregiver. Much to my surprise, she responded that she would be willing to serve in that role. She was also still going to give us the family discount by only charging ten dollars an hour. This was truly an answer to prayer, and the gratitude I felt was immeasurable. However, she did ask that we give her two weeks advance notice before Mom's release so she could adjust her schedule with her other clients.

Daniel had also decided to move in with Mom. Although he lived next door and could get to her quickly, we all agreed that someone needed to be in the home with her at night so there would be no delays in case she needed help. I don't think Daniel could ever realize the extent of the gratitude my siblings and I felt for his selflessness. We certainly didn't take it for granted. Despite how badly Mom had treated him over the last couple of years, he hadn't hesitated to step up to do what was needed to allow her to come home and keep her safe. She just needed to get stronger.

At 5:40 p.m., while resting at home, I noticed that I had forgotten to turn my phone's ringer back on. I had a message from my niece, Leigh, who was visiting Mom at the hospital. When I retrieved the message, it was Mom's voice that I heard. She said, "LaBena I've been kidnapped, and I am being held hostage. Do whatever you have to do to get me back because I'm scared. Be careful because I don't want you to get kidnapped, too."

I immediately called Leigh, who said Mom was agitated and thought Leigh was one of her captors. Understandably, she was shaken, having never seen my mom in such a state. I assured her that Mom was experiencing delusions because of her illnesses and instructed Leigh to have the nurses get a doctor to order something to calm her down, which she did. However, Mom refused the medications. When I asked Leigh if she felt I should return to the hospital, she said no. She said she would stay with Mom until she calmed down and would call me with an update once she left the hospital.

About an hour later, Leigh called to let me know Mom had taken her medication and had settled down. She no longer thought Leigh was a captor, thinking instead she had been kidnapped as well. Mom told Leigh to tell me to stay away because she didn't want me to be kidnapped. Leigh also said that the hospital was going to provide a sitter to stay with Mom through the night. I planned to go back the next day

(Monday), so I was fine with that. After hanging up, I called each of my brothers to relay the happenings of the day, leaving it up to them to decide whether they wanted to venture back to the hospital.

When I arrived at the hospital, I was met at Mom's door by a young nursing student from Kent State University who had been sitting with Mom that morning. "Your mom has been very talkative and pleasant. She has been speaking about her time as an employee at Kent State," she said. Mom had worked as a cook at Kent State University in the sixties and often spoke of how much she enjoyed interacting with the students. I was surprised to learn that Mom had remembered and shared the different locations she had worked and explained which were her favorites. The student also stated that Mom had been speaking about her children and would be happy to see me. Unfortunately, the person the young student had described to me was not the person I saw when I entered the room.

Resting on her side, Mom did not look up, and did not speak. Instead, I watched as a slow stream of tears fell from her eyes, across her nose, down her cheek, and onto her pillow. I stroked her head and asked what was wrong, but she wouldn't respond. Being the crybaby that I am, the tears began streaming down my face as well. Mom looked so sad. It just broke my heart. I knew Mom was where she needed to be, but I rarely saw her cry. This was too much to bear! It was then that I began to believe that my mom was dying, not actively, but nonetheless dying. I was on an emotional rollercoaster and could only imagine what Mom was feeling.

Finally, Mom looked up at me and asked, "What is wrong with me?" I told her about the various diagnosed infections (which now included emphysema) and stressed the importance of taking medications and cooperating with the physical therapists so she could get stronger and go home. I had developed a habit of always speaking to Mom as if she were lucid. If there was a chance that she could understand what I was saying, I wanted to ensure I was speaking at her pre-dementia level.

She then became more talkative and shared her kidnapping story with me. "I need you to be very careful. I don't want you to be kidnapped like I was. They tie you up, take you to this place, and stick things in you. They don't give you what you want, and they get mad at you when you don't eat what they give you." As I tried to reason with her, I remembered more of the dementia rules.

> **Lesson:** Join them in their reality instead of trying to bring them into yours.

I let her know I was sorry for what she was going through and would do whatever I could to help her. She was satisfied with my response and relaxed.

Whenever Daniel had a break in his schedule, he dropped by to check on Mom. He took care of any need she had at that given time, not wanting her to have to wait for someone else to assist her. I would fuss at him, stating that he should let others do their jobs. His response was always the same: "If I am here and she needs something done, I will take care of it. I am not going to have her wait for what she needs if I can handle it." He was so devoted to her.

We learned that Mom was scheduled to be released from Central Hospital in the next couple of days. As such, we needed to decide whether she would be returning to Cedar Glen. Daniel and I again reviewed the list of facilities that accepted Medicare, although I don't know why. Nothing had changed since the last time we reviewed the list. Daniel was still legally blind and unable to drive, and there were still only two facilities that accepted Medicare. In the end, the decision was made to have her return to Cedar Glen. The stipulation for this return was that she be placed in a single room as opposed to sharing a room with a roommate. Because of the contagious nature of her infections, the facility had no problem accommodating our request this time.

105

And take the helmet of salvation, and the sword of the Spirit, which is the word of God: Praying with all prayer and supplication in the Spirit, and watching thereunto with all perseverance and supplication for all saints. Ephesians 6:17–18

Chapter 16
Rehab: Round Three

Monday morning, Daniel called to say that Mom was being returned to Cedar Glen later that day. I was alarmed, to say the least. Mom was now actively battling pneumonia, sepsis (Healthline.com states that "Sepsis is a life-threatening illness caused by your body's response to an infection"), *C. diff*, VRE, emphysema, and her original UTI. How could she be returning to rehab? What were they thinking? I was surprised that Cedar Glen would take her back with so much going on. I guess money is money!

I informed Daniel that I couldn't come out that particular day because I had to pick up Ann from school but assured him that I would be out bright and early on Tuesday. He told me that he had taken the week off work, so he would be available for the transfer and could spend time with her afterward. He later called to let me know that the transfer had gone well, Mom had her private room, and the same safety protocols that were in place at the hospital were in place at the rehab facility. I had to mentally prepare myself for the gloves, gown, mask, and the idea of not touching my mom.

When I arrived on Tuesday, Daniel was already in the room. Mom was sitting up in her wheelchair (which had been provided in an attempt to eliminate her back pain while sitting), eating lunch and looking out of the window. She seemed genuinely happy to see me, asking about my husband and the Little Squirt, a.k.a. my granddaughter, Ann. I was thrilled to see that she seemed to be re-acclimating to the facility.

Mom began to speak of her kidnapping again. I smiled and she became angry. She told me that she hoped it never happened to me because she didn't want me to see how it feels. She began asking me to hide different items from her food tray because she would get into trouble if she didn't eat it. She said her kidnappers would poke her with things, fuss at her, and tell her they would put things in her if she didn't eat. Suddenly, I had a lightbulb moment.

Mom had been seriously ill, feverish, and nonresponsive. Strangers had entered her home, Cedar Glen, wrapped her in blankets, put her on a gurney, placed her in the back of a vehicle, and taken her to an unfamiliar location. When she arrived at that location, people took off her clothes, began sticking needles and IVs into her, and began fussing at her. In her mind, the paramedics were her kidnappers. It all made perfect sense now. She *had* been kidnapped! She was being held against her will. She was confused, but not delusional. It was quite amazing to think of how she'd made the mental connections.

Lesson: Look for the truths in what may appear to be nonsensical. It may not be nonsense at all.

Mom continued to look out of the window with a huge smile on her face. When I asked what she was looking at, she said that she was looking at the horse. "What horse?" I asked. She said, "Don't you see that horse out there? You have to be blind not to see it." I told her again that I didn't see a horse and attempted to see if there was anything outside that vaguely resembled a horse. There wasn't.

Mom was becoming agitated because I didn't see what she was seeing. "LaBena, you can't see that horse? Look. It's right there." "Oh. I see it now," I said. Mom responded, "I was just about to tell you to clean your glasses because I don't know how you couldn't see that big old thing." I began to wonder if her hallucination was because of the dementia or because she was nearing the end of life. Having sat vigil with many hospice patients, I knew that hallucinations and visions were common as they neared death.

On this day, Mom did not mention going home. Physically, she seemed much better so I would have expected home to be a constant topic of conversation. However, I was very grateful it wasn't.

108

I hadn't realized the toll that the back and forth had taken on me. Although my treatment for Lyme disease was going well, it felt as if my body were beginning to shut down. I was having severe stomach pains and headaches. I knew myself well enough to know that the stress of the past few weeks was about to cause a physical crash. I needed to take a few steps back and take time to replenish myself. Although I wanted to continue to visit Mom, I had to take a break and allow myself some time to mend. I prayed for a quick healing as I succumbed to a stomach virus. Fortunately, healing came quickly for me. After about four days, I was ready to resume my trips to see Mom.

Lesson: You can't adequately care for others if you don't take care of yourself. Put your own oxygen mask on first.

I missed seeing Mom and was anxious to go for a visit. My brothers had been diligent in visiting her daily. They were such good sons! They shared that she had been putting major guilt trips on them. "After everything I've done for you this is how you treat me," she would say continually. I had not yet experienced that with her and was glad. It was hard for them to hear her say those words. I tried to break up the tension by reminding them that she once told me she had so many kids (seven) so there'd be someone to take care of her when she got old. That always brought about a laugh.

On my way to the SNF, I decided to pick up a couple of Mom's favorite foods: fried chicken wings and coleslaw from KFC. When I arrived, I put on the required protective gear and entered Mom's room. An aide was sitting on her bed, trying to convince her to get into it. The aide said that Mom was tired and wanted to go to bed, but she wanted *her* bed. When I asked Mom if she'd like to eat before getting into bed, she said no. Again, she stated she wanted her bed.

I let her know that I had brought her wings and coleslaw for lunch, but she was having none of it. She wanted to go home to her bed and nothing else was going to satisfy her. As I thought more about it, I couldn't blame her. Her bed was fluffy and comfortable, not like the hard hospital-style beds that were common in rehab facilities. I'd want my own bed too!

Knowing that was not possible, I advised her that our goal was to get her back to her home and her own bed but that she just wasn't well enough yet. If she continued to take her medications and do what she was being asked to do, she would be able to go home soon. She looked at me and asked, "You swear?" That shocked me. She had never asked anything like that before. I responded that our goal was for her to go home and that we were putting measures in place for her to get home; Daniel had taken the week off work to make sure her home was like it needed to be once she returned, and she just needed to get stronger.

Mom was satisfied with my response and agreed to get into bed. What I was not prepared for was the way she screamed while reclining. I know the complaints of pain had become the norm, but I wasn't expecting the scream, and it unnerved me. The aide told me that they had recently given her something for pain and that it should kick in shortly. Soon the pain meds provided the desired relief, and Mom was resting comfortably.

As I stood to go place Mom's lunch in the fridge, she cried out, "You are not leaving me alone here, are you?" I told her I was just going to refrigerate her food, but she didn't want me to go. She told me she was scared and asked me not to leave. When I asked what she was afraid of, she said, "I don't know." I sat back down, and she relaxed.

Mom closed her eyes but did not go to sleep. Occasionally, she opened them and asked, "Are they paying you to stay with me?" At first, I asked her why she thought I was being paid to sit with her. Then I realized that my mom didn't always know who I was. As heartbreaking as that was, I couldn't take it personally. I just needed to treasure those moments when she did know me. I was still saddened as I thought about what was to come.

Mom asked for Daniel throughout my visit. She wanted to know if he was in the building, where he was, and when he would be coming to visit. I let her know that he would come as soon as he got off work and that he'd want her to rest.

At one point, Mom looked at the wall and appeared very frightened. When I asked what she was looking at, she said she was watching the shadows of the men chasing each other and she was scared. I turned the lights out so she wouldn't see shadows. I made a mental note to tell her physician that she was hallucinating and that what she was seeing was frightening to her. They would need to give her something to curtail her terrors.

After a while, Mom looked at me and said, "I'm not going home, am I?" I assured her that our goal was for her to go back to her home. I reminded her that we had already put some things in place for her and that she'd be going home as soon as she was stronger. She was okay in that moment, but I wasn't. I was becoming more convinced that Mom had a limited time on this earth, and that thought made my heart hurt.

Mom announced that she had to go to the restroom, so I called for an aide to assist her. When the aide arrived, she asked if we were from Detroit and said that Mom had spent a great deal of time speaking about Detroit earlier that day. I had been born in Detroit in 1954 but had no memories of my time spent there. I decided that I should bring a notebook to keep in Mom's room so people could communicate things that she would say.

Right after Mom had returned to bed, Daniel showed up. Mom's face lit up like a lightbulb when she saw him, and then she sat up and announced that she was hungry. I teased Daniel about being the favorite child, a position once held by Nicholas, letting him know Mom had been asking for him all day. He smiled and told me that Mom always asked for me when I wasn't around. "Sure she does," I said. Daniel then gave me a lesson on what could and could not be done regarding the food I'd brought, and scolded me for not following isolation protocol because I had hugged Mom.

111

I explained that I was adhering to it more than Mom's hands-on caregivers, and I couldn't help but hug her if I saw she was upset. He said that the reason Mom was in the shape she was in was probably because caregivers had not been following protocol, and that we needed to gently remind them to wear gowns and gloves when caring for her. I told him that was fine, but they had shared that wearing of gloves and gowns was optional for them. When I heard that, I agreed with Daniel that their lack of following protocol may have been responsible not only for Mom's illness, but also the illnesses of other residents.

Lesson: When interviewing potential facilities for your loved ones, ask what protocols are in place for working with residents with contagious illnesses, and whether staff adherence to those protocols is mandatory.

As Mom ate the food I had brought for her, I said my goodbyes and began walking towards the door. "When are you coming back?" she asked. I responded that I would be returning in a couple of days, and she was satisfied with that response. I smiled.

I made plans to attend my mom's care conference the following Tuesday, during which the social worker, nursing supervisor, and physical therapist would discuss the progress of each patient and future strategies for continued improvement. During Mom's meeting, everyone stated that she did extremely well when she chose to do so. When I asked what that meant, they informed me that when Mom was in a bad mood, she would be uncooperative, and when she was in a good mood, she'd do very well. According to them, her progress was contingent upon her attitude. That sounded normal to me.

I asked them to share what improvements they had seen regarding her physical capabilities. They said she could walk thirty feet and navigate stairs with the assistance of a walker, but that she still required moderate to major assistance with activities of daily living (ADLs). One of their major concerns continued to be cognitive deficiencies. Mom had very poor judgment, and safety was a concern. Mom would continuously forget that she couldn't stand independently and was a huge fall risk. She had fallen multiple times at Cedar Glen and at the hospital. Falls typically occurred when she would try to get up to go to the restroom.

This comment frustrated me because I had suggested that staff check on her hourly for toileting. Despite that suggestion, their solution was to have her use her call button if she needed to get up. She had dementia. She was not going to remember to use a call button; she couldn't even remember what a call button was. My takeaway was that there needed to be a rehab facility that was specific to persons with dementia, and that it needed to be sufficiently staffed to serve that population. Cedar Glen was not adequately staffed to meet Mom's needs. I didn't believe any *regular* rehab facility could meet her needs.

I asked when they thought Mom would be going home, and they provided a timeframe of two weeks. They also stressed the importance of her not being left alone—ever—because of her poor judgment. I let them know that we'd already arranged for a full-time caregiver to be with Mom during the day, and that Daniel would be with her in the evenings.

Before ending the care conference, we discussed what equipment would be needed at home. The physical therapist and occupational therapist both recommended a wheelchair, a bedside commode, an elevated toilet seat, and a walker. They asked what other equipment I thought would be needed. I had no idea and asked if they could do an in-home assessment and make recommendations based upon what they saw. They agreed that an in-home assessment was a good idea and scheduled it for the following Thursday.

Despite my anxiety about Mom's coming home, I was happy that we at least had a target date for her return—especially since a week ago I didn't see that happening. Even though Mom wouldn't remember, we could share that information with her. If she asked about going home, we could give her a timeframe as opposed to just telling her, "When you get stronger." That would make her happy . . . for the moment.

Daniel had already made some modifications to the home. All living room furniture had been elevated, with special attention to Mom's recliner. Rails were placed where they were needed, and excess clutter removed. All preliminary preparation had been completed.

On Thursday, when the occupational therapist arrived at Mom's home, she noted the twelve steps Mom had to climb to get from the garage to her living room. She tested the handrails for sturdiness and stated they were great. She asked how frequently we expected Mom to use those stairs, and I told her that I didn't expect her to use them at all once she got home. She assessed all other key areas and made recommendations for modifications and equipment.

After the assessment, I went through Mom's clothing, removing items that I knew were too large or too small, as well as those that appeared dirty or stained. I intended to take the soiled clothes to my home to see if they could be cleaned, discard those that were not salvageable, and bag the rest to give away. While going through the clothes, I came across a dress that Mom had worn to the wedding of one of her grandchildren. It was a beautiful, pale blue chiffon dress with tiny silver sequins fashioned throughout the bodice. It also had long sleeves, which were important to Mom because she was always cold. I remembered how much she loved the dress and her saying that she'd probably never have another opportunity to wear it.

As I was recalling her comment, I felt as though I heard a voice telling me that she'd wear it one more time. It was so strong and eerily real that I decided to take the dress and have it professionally cleaned. I learned long ago to trust those feelings when they were so strong.

After loading up my car with the clothing, I decided to fix Mom some lunch. Unfortunately, I took longer than intended working on the clothes and was fearful that she would have already eaten by the time I reached Cedar Glen. I arrived, with piping hot fried green tomatoes in hand, right after Mom had finished eating lunch; however, that did not stop her from enjoying her tomatoes. She reached out for the plate they were on and ate every single one. It warmed my heart to see how much she enjoyed them, and I was glad I had taken the time to prepare them for her.

She thanked me for the tomatoes and told me how good they were. It was the most I'd seen her eat in quite a while. She had become very particular about what she ate, almost childlike. She liked what she liked, and wouldn't try anything that she felt she wouldn't, or didn't like. Who knew that fried green tomatoes would bring her so much joy? I decided I would prepare them for her again on the day she returned home.

During the visit, Mom was pleasant. She asked about George, Lynn, Yvonne, and Ann. She smiled, laughed, and was extremely talkative. She told me she was surprised and happy to see me because she was lonely. I don't recall Mom ever telling me she was lonely. That broke my heart.

Years ago, following her initial time in rehab, she had spent many days alone in her home. During all that time, she never once mentioned being lonely. She had gone from driving and going wherever she wanted to being virtually confined to her home. Granted, my brothers and I had jobs and/or families and were not able to visit often during the week, but I still felt guilty and wondered if there was more we could have done for her. Of course there was, but hindsight is twenty-twenty.

When I got home, I had the feeling that I needed to begin writing Mom's obituary. I didn't question what I was feeling. I just grabbed my computer and began typing.

Later that evening, I called Daniel to discuss the recommendations that had been made during the in-home assessment. We didn't have too much to do. It was just a matter of performing a final check of supplies and equipment, doing the grocery shopping, and seeing if the caregiver would have a problem caring for Mom while she had *C. diff.*

I contacted Meisha, who assured me that she'd had to deal with that issue endless times in the past and that it would not be a problem for her. I confirmed Mom's homecoming date, thanked her, and let her know we would have gowns, gloves, and anything else she felt she needed. We also discussed protocols for providing care, and cleaning precautions. I knew that Meisha was more than aware of what needed to be done, but felt that discussing it would avoid any future misunderstandings.

I was concerned about the contagiousness of *C. diff* and the fact that Mom's home only had one restroom. Although Mom would have a bedside commode, waste would still be disposed of in the restroom and put anyone who used it at high risk for contracting *C. diff*. We needed to be extremely careful when disposing of waste and when cleaning.

From what Daniel had shared with me and what I'd read on my own, the spores of *C. diff* needed to be avoided. Spores are found in feces and urine, and bleach is the only effective method of getting rid of them. In addition, not all disinfecting wipes are effective, so I became an expert at reading the labels. After searching for what we needed, I decided to stick with good old-fashioned bleach!

Lesson: All disinfecting wipes are not created equal. Read the labels to ensure that what you are purchasing will do what you need it to do.

The two weeks leading up to Mom's return home passed very quickly. On the Friday before her scheduled release from Cedar Glen, I arranged for my brothers to meet me there to put plans in place. We met in the facility's living room, where Mom was already sitting and picking at her dinner.

We discussed grocery shopping. In the past, Nicholas, Don, and I had taken turns taking Mom and Daniel shopping on Saturday mornings. Since Mom was no longer able to go due to her physical limitations and was unable to be left home alone, two of us needed to be available on shopping days. One person would need to stay with Mom as the other took Daniel shopping for both himself and Mom.

I could tell Daniel was troubled by this. He'd always felt like he was a bother, but that was far from the case. We were all grateful for everything he was doing for Mom and were more than fine with assisting him with whatever he needed. My biggest concern was, and had always been, that he wouldn't let us know when he needed help. We had to be sure that we showed up, as opposed to asking whether he needed assistance. We knew Daniel liked to work out after work, so coming to keep an eye on Mom during that time would be a great help to him, we thought.

After telling my brothers that I would continue to come out multiple times during the week, we agreed that on my assigned afternoon (when the caregiver would work only half a day), I would spend the night. That evening would be the perfect time for grocery shopping since I would already be there keeping an eye on Mom. Our plan was complete, and everyone agreed. I thought about how fortunate we were to have all of us on the same page, trying to do what was best for Mom. That was truly a blessing.

Throughout our meeting, Mom kept repeating, "I'm ready to go now." We told her she would be going home on the following day. We let her know that we would pick her up after her supplies were delivered and after she ate lunch. She would be complacent for a little while, only to shout, "Can we go now?" a few moments later.

We all stayed with Mom until she was ready for bed and got her settled in. We were happy that she would be going home because that's all she desired. By the same token, we were deeply concerned because the *C. diff* was in full force. She was incontinent and still falling because she couldn't remember she was unable to walk and would attempt to get up and go to the restroom.

Imagine this poor woman throwing her legs over the bolster that is meant to keep her from falling out of bed, trying to stand up, and crashing to the floor. We later learned the full extent of the damage caused by her falls at home, out with friends (which we hadn't known about), in the hospital, and at Cedar Glen.

I gathered her things (except for what she would need on Saturday), placed them in plastic bags, and said my goodbyes. I washed everything immediately at Mom's in the hopes of avoiding any cross contamination. I planned to stay overnight so Daniel and I could address any last-minute needs, and was doubtful either one of us would get much sleep as we anticipated Mom's return home.

Is any among you afflicted? Let him pray. Is any merry? Let him sing psalms. Is any sick among you? Let him call for the elders of the church; and let them pray over him, anointing him with oil in the name of the Lord. And the prayer of faith shall save the sick, and the Lord shall raise him up; and if he have committed sins, they shall be forgiven him. James 5:13–15

Chapter 17
There is No Place Like Home

Daniel and I had planned pretty much everything: how to get Mom into and out of my SUV, how to get her up those twelve steps, and what to prepare for dinner. We even had her favorite chair set up so she could sit and look out of the window at the birds, a beloved pastime. But, of course, things did not go as planned.

When we went to get Mom, she was sitting in a wheelchair near the nurse's station. Although her lunch tray was resting in front of her, she had barely eaten. She was ready to go, and her face lit up like a lightbulb when she saw us. The nurse approached Daniel to make him aware that all of Mom's medications were in the bag she was handing him, and to tell him which ones had already been administered. She then told us that we needed to schedule a follow-up appointment with Mom's primary care physician for one week after her release from Cedar Glen and went on her way.

I suggested that Mom attempt to go to the restroom prior to our leaving the facility. She said she didn't need to go but would try. Unfortunately, she didn't make it to the restroom and was wearing the only clothes we had left for her. Because she lived so close, I was able to quickly go pick up more clothing and return to get her. By the time I returned, she had been cleaned up and was ready to don the fresh clothing I had retrieved. I threw the soiled clothing away, not even wanting to deal with the idea of trying to get them cleaned without being exposed to the *C. diff* spores.

I witnessed how impulsive Mom's behavior was. She exercised no judgment. Moving quickly and recklessly, she almost fell getting back into her wheelchair. I became increasingly anxious thinking about this new adventure we were about to embark upon. Would Meisha, who was as small as Mom, be able to handle her and adequately care for her? Was this going to work? Was Mom ready to come home? These questions—

and more—continued to whirl in my mind as we moved Mom towards my vehicle.

Mom was extremely attentive during the ride home, taking in all her surroundings. As we pulled into her driveway she asked, "Whose house is this?" I was taken aback at the idea that she didn't recognize her own home. This home she had been craving for weeks was now foreign to her. "This is your home, Mom," I said. She became quiet, and I wondered what she was thinking. She did not utter another word for quite some time.

Daniel got Mom out of my SUV and into the wheelchair, but with quite a bit of effort. Mom seemed to have difficulty following his simple instructions: "Grab the bar with your left hand . . . Move your right foot . . . Put your arms around my waist . . . Grab my arm . . ." Although each command was given separately to allow ample time for compliance, she just couldn't seem to handle the requests. It took a long time to get her into that wheelchair, and my anxiety increased with each attempted task.

As I peered at the steps she needed to navigate, I reminded myself to breathe. Could she climb the twelve steps required to reach the living room, or would Daniel need to carry her? The physical therapist had said she would have no problem, but I was not so sure.

Eight minutes later, we reached the top. Mom hadn't ascended those steps quickly in years, but prior to her last fall at home, it may have taken her three minutes or less to climb the steps independently. Not now, and perhaps never again.

We had placed a chair at the top of the stairs, anticipating that she would be tired once she reached the top, but tired was an understatement. She was exhausted! I was witnessing a decline and could not understand why it was happening so rapidly. Her favorite chair was less than three steps away, but she did not want to sit in it. She wanted to go to bed.

Daniel placed a walker in front of her and helped her get situated with it. She didn't move. Why wasn't she moving? He began giving her literal, step-by-step instructions that she seemed unable to follow.

"Mom, move your feet," he said. She attempted to move them, but they weren't cooperating. If, according to her physical therapist, she was taking thirty steps with a walker, why wasn't she walking now? Perhaps she had forgotten how.

After what seemed like an eternity, she began to move. We were now standing before the three steps she needed to climb to get to her bedroom from the living room. Again, Daniel provided instructions, but almost ended up climbing the steps for her. I could see his disappointment at her lack of ability to perform what seemed like simple tasks, especially since we had been told that she was able to do them. Although I'd visited during different times of the day, she was always resting when I arrived. I realized that I had never seen Mom perform any of the tasks I had been informed she could perform.

Lesson: Ask for the evidence instead of believing what you are told.

A second walker, which included a seat, was at the top of the steps leading to Mom's bedroom. When she reached the top of the steps, Daniel had her sit on the walker seat and rolled her to the bed she had been begging for since her first night away. I was so happy to see her return to her bed but was saddened by her visible weakness. I fought back tears as we helped her get changed and maneuvered her into her beloved bed. Was she truly ready to be home?

I thought back to a few months ago when I felt as though God had told me Mom would not be alive for her April 2nd birthday. Today was March 17. Would she be able to hold on for sixteen more days? She was a fighter who would always rally when people thought she wouldn't make it. I did not want to lose my mom, but I also hated her diminished quality of life. I was amazed she was able to bear the weight of all she had been carrying.

As soon as Mom was settled into bed she went to sleep, so Daniel and I went downstairs to review her medications and to get things organized for Meisha, who would be coming on board full-time in two days. Matching the medications to the list we were provided proved to be a daunting task. It turned out we had received items that were not on the medication list and had not received some items that were on the list. I organized the medications by the times and frequency they were to be taken, but then backtracked because I didn't understand why she was on some of them.

We had been given four different medications for the treatment of hypertension. I reflected on her last hospitalization, when her blood pressure was extremely high and they had trouble lowering it, and my last rehab visit when I felt her blood pressure was low. I had requested a consultation with the physician who was monitoring her, but he never seemed to be around when I was in the facility. He also never called me as I requested. I should have been more persistent.

Daniel called the Cedar Glen nurse to ask about the medications. One of the missing medications was an over the counter probiotic. Another was an antibiotic that had been provided in case a recent urinalysis came back positive for a UTI. The nurse had thought she put it in the bag, but it wasn't there. There was another medication we were told had been discontinued. She then provided Daniel with the rationale behind each of the hypertension medications Mom was taking and said we should continue with them until we met with the primary care physician.

I was especially intrigued by the idea that we had been provided medication for breathing treatments. Neither Daniel nor I had ever witnessed Mom receiving a breathing treatment although, having emphysema and pneumonia, it seemed more than appropriate. We were told it was there in case we needed it. Sigh!

I went back to Cedar Glen to retrieve the missing antibiotic for the probable UTI and was given only two doses. I was told that the pharmacy had not sent the rest of the medication and that it would need to be picked up in a couple of days if Mom's test came back positive. I didn't make a big deal about it since Daniel worked nearby and would easily be able to come by to pick up the antibiotic if needed.

Next, I went to a local pharmacy to secure the probiotic she had been prescribed. I was actually happy to learn that she had been prescribed this medication. From my own experience with Lyme disease and the amount of time I'd taken antibiotics, I knew they could kill both good and bad bacteria. The probiotics would repopulate the intestines with good bacteria and hopefully counteract the damage being done by *C. diff* and the antibiotics.

Using a large whiteboard that Daniel had purchased, I created a medication chart with each medication, why it was being given, and when it was to be given. Daniel then prepared the appropriate pillboxes with medications to be administered at certain times of day. We wanted to do as much as possible to ensure that we, and Meisha, would be properly medicating Mom. Because we had to rely on Meisha to give the medications throughout the day, we wanted to lessen the potential for errors.

Next, Daniel and I reviewed the list of caregiver responsibilities I had previously typed up, made necessary revisions, and called Meisha with an update to ensure all was set for her to begin working on Monday. Lastly, I put our caregiver journal in place. It would serve as our communication log, with Daniel and me leaving written instructions and information for Meisha, and Meisha providing important feedback to us. It was also a place for her to record when she gave Mom her medications and what she had given her.

Lesson: When multiple persons are caring for a loved one at home, timely and accurate communication is crucial. A care journal is an excellent tool for everyone to read and record in it when they visit. It is also useful for tracking behaviors and what may have precipitated those behaviors. The journal can accompany you on doctor visits as well.

I planned to stay at Mom's for the day, but Daniel convinced me to go home. He was fairly confident that she would sleep for the remainder of the day, so there was no need for me to stay. Agreeing, I went home.

Of course, I called Daniel on Sunday to see how things were going, and he stated that she wasn't eating and was quiet. He was not sure that she realized she was at home, and we both found that interesting. For a month she had been requesting to return to a place that she now could not recognize.

At 8:00 a.m. on Monday morning, Meisha showed up as planned. Before leaving for work, Daniel had time to give her a quick tour of the home and give her instructions. We had previously planned to do this when Mom came home on Saturday, but something had come up with another client and Meisha was unable to come by. She had my number and knew she was to call me with any questions or concerns, so we didn't anticipate any problems.

Mom was still lethargic on Monday, so she was fairly easy to handle . . . except for her explosive diarrhea. She was not eating and taking only a few sips of water, according to Meisha. I asked her to track Mom's bowel movements and fluid intake in the care journal so I could relay that information to the physician during her scheduled appointment on Friday. Considering the difficulty she had had when coming home, I was concerned about trying to transport her to the doctor and decided to call a transport company for the trip. A visiting nurse was scheduled to come by on Thursday, so I planned to discuss this further with her at that time.

Meisha called at the end of the day and reported all info from her time with Mom. She had spent most of the day doing laundry because of Mom's *C. diff* issues, but there was nothing else crucial at that time. She remained with Mom until Daniel arrived home, briefly updated him, and left for the day. Tuesday did not go as well.

Mom was more alert on Tuesday and did not like the idea of Meisha, or anyone else, being in her home. I'd anticipated this, so it was no surprise. Meisha called me when she couldn't get Mom to take her scheduled medications. I asked her to give Mom the phone, and I tried to convince Mom to take her meds. Unfortunately, she was having no part of it. She wanted this woman out of her house and was not going to take any medication from her. Because I did not want to bother Daniel at work, I told Meisha I would call Don and ask him to come over to see if he could get Mom to take her medication.

About forty minutes later Meisha called to say that Don had come over and was able to get Mom to take her medication. In addition to the scheduled medications, I suggested that Don give her antianxiety medication. That settled her down and she was much calmer the remainder of the afternoon. Unfortunately, Mom's diarrhea continued to be a concern.

Wednesday was pretty much a repeat of Tuesday, except Mom took most of her scheduled medications without problems. I wasn't concerned when she refused one of her supplements. I knew her numbers were good for that particular mineral, so I told Meisha not to worry about it.

Meisha again expressed that Mom was having quite a bit of diarrhea; as a result, she was spending most of her time doing laundry and cleaning. Mom was still not eating and taking only a few sips of water. She had to be close to becoming dehydrated if she wasn't already. Daniel would be home soon and could determine if Mom had any additional needs. I was scheduled to come out the following day and could relay our concerns to the visiting nurse at that time.

After I arrived on Thursday morning and received the updates from Meisha, I went to Mom's room and was very concerned by what I saw. Mom was beyond lethargic. When I called her name, she opened her eyes and immediately closed them. She did not respond to any questions or comments, and her hands felt very warm. I asked Meisha if she had heard anything from the visiting nurse regarding when she would be arriving, and she had not.

When I called the nurse's office, the receptionist stated that the nurse had called us three times, and no one had answered the phone. Owed a confirmation call the previous day, I knew that neither Daniel nor I had received a call or a message from the nurse. I was becoming agitated and needed to take a step back to calm myself down.

I told the receptionist that I needed to have a nurse visit that day; not coming was not an option. I told her my mom was scheduled to see her physician on Friday, but I was sure we would not be able to transport her in her present condition. "I'll have the nurse call you," she said. I went to check on Mom, whose condition hadn't changed. I felt she was dehydrated and was hoping the nurse could give her an IV to hydrate her.

The nurse, Mindy, called and restated that she had called three times. When I asked why she hadn't left a message, she said the voicemail had not been set up. It was then that I knew she had called the wrong number. Upon checking, there was an incorrect digit in the number she had been given. I couldn't understand how that occurred since both occupational therapy and physical therapy had been able to reach us to schedule their appointments for the following week. Why was the phone number she had different from theirs when they all worked for the same company?

According to Mindy, she had been in Ravenna that morning and would not be back because she was headed to Ashtabula. I let her know that was not acceptable. Sometimes you have to push a little harder to get your desired result. I had a great deal of experience being assertive while being respectful, but I also knew how to bring out the B-card if necessary. I was hoping it would not be. I let her know that the fact she had been given an incorrect phone number by her staff was not my concern and that I expected Mom to be seen that day as planned.

When she asked what my concern was, I shared that information with her. She then told me that it was probably a good idea to take Mom to the ER. I told Mindy that I expected that she come and assess Mom. I didn't want to have Mom moved unless it was deemed necessary because I knew how upsetting it would be for her. Mindy then stated that she would be at Mom's house within the hour. That was more like it!

Mindy arrived in half an hour, which surprised and pleased me. She assessed Mom and determined that her pulse ox reading (the percentage of oxygen saturation in the blood) and blood pressure were both low, and that she was indeed dehydrated. She made a call to Mom's primary physician, who recommended that we take her to the ER. We were all in agreement.

I called EMS because I knew I would not be able to transport her. I thanked Mindy for coming, and she asked me to text her to let her know the outcome of the ER visit. Now it was time to tell my brothers what was going on and wait for the ambulance.

The thought of repeating that whole cycle of hospital to rehab made me sick in the pit of my stomach. Mom would be so sad.

Thy kingdom come. Thy will be done in earth, as it is in heaven. Give us this day our daily bread. Matthew 6:10–11

Chapter 18
I Don't Want to Go

When I let Mom know that we had to go to the hospital, she said softly, "I don't want to go," but offered no resistance. That concerned me. She was quiet as the paramedics got her onto the cot, down the stairs, and into the ambulance. This made me realize how ill she was.

I followed the ambulance to the hospital, and it occurred to me that this would be the first time I would be the one waiting alone in the ER. Daniel and Nicholas were at work, and I didn't feel there was a reason for them to leave at that point. They would just be waiting while tests were being run, and there was nothing for them to do. Don's daughter, Veda, was having surgery for a brain aneurism, so I didn't want to call him unless it was absolutely necessary. I opted to send everyone texts apprising them of what was happening and assuring them that I would continue to provide updates.

I found myself trying to pray, but I wasn't sure what to pray for. Was I supposed to pray for healing for my almost ninety-year-old mom? Would that be selfish? Was I supposed to ask God to take her out of her misery? Would that be cruel? I could continue to pray for my niece, asking that her surgery go well. I settled on the Lord's Prayer. After all, isn't that the prayer Jesus told us to pray: "For your Father knoweth what things ye have need of, before ye ask Him." That would work!

After about two hours, I looked up and saw a woman wearing scrubs approaching me. I could tell from the look on her face that she was not looking forward to what she was about to tell me. I instantly knew that the dreaded H-word was about to be spoken. The woman was a nurse practitioner. She sat across from me, confirmed my identity, and said, "I am about to ask some questions and say some things that I hope you won't view as insensitive."

I decided to put her out of her misery by saying, "You want to talk to me about hospice, don't you?" I told her it was okay because it was something I knew was coming. She then proceeded to review Mom's most recent hospital admissions and discuss the toll her infections were taking on her body. The infections were becoming more difficult for Mom to fight off and were leaving her weaker with each occurrence. "How aggressive do you want us to be?" she asked.

I responded that my brothers and I would need to have some discussion to decide what we should do. She shared the tests that had been ordered and said I would be able to see Mom soon. I thanked her and she walked away. Settling into my own thoughts, I was again fighting back tears. I suddenly felt alone and thought that this must have been how Daniel felt during his many times alone in the ER. Daniel was much stronger than I. After just one time, I knew I didn't want to experience this ever again.

It was about 5:30 p.m. before I was finally allowed to see Mom. Walking toward the area where she was being held, I reflected on the last time I made that walk and began to prepare myself for what I was about to see. Daniel had gotten off work and was already sitting with Mom. Isolation protocols were in place, so I put on protective gear before entering her room. Unlike last time, she was still and quiet, not fussing when people provided care. Was this cause for alarm?

After another hour or two, we looked up to see the nurse practitioner who had spoken with me earlier, and the same ER physician we had seen during our last visit. They looked somber, and I was sure that they were about to give us some devastating news. I said, "I don't think you are going to tell us anything that will surprise us. Please just say what you need to say."

They mentioned Mom's frailness and I began zoning in and out of the conversation. "Blah, blah, blah . . . infection. Blah, blah, blah . . . frail. Blah, blah, blah . . . recurring. Blah, blah, blah . . . advanced directives. Blah, blah, blah . . . CPR." I was listening, but not hearing. I

129

didn't want to hear. Although I knew where we were headed, I truly was not ready to go there.

Before they entered the room, Daniel had asked if I felt we should begin to focus on comfort care from now on. I could only imagine how difficult it was for him to utter those words. He was so dedicated to Mom and loved her unconditionally. His loss would be greater than all of ours because he had spent so much more time with her. We could try to say that we would all feel the same as Daniel, but we wouldn't. He had accepted the inevitable. "I agree," I said.

The physician and nurse practitioner were now asking us to make that same decision. They asked, "How would you like us to proceed?" I responded that my siblings and I would need to meet and discuss the next steps. We needed to see how Don and Nicholas were feeling about everything, and I wasn't sure when that meeting would take place. When they stated that they would consult with the admitting physician to see whether Mom could be admitted to the hospital, I blurted, "You will admit her." The nurse practitioner, somewhat shocked, replied, "That was a pretty forceful response." I apologized. Having been there for close to eight hours, I was tired, sad, cranky, and frightened. That, however, did not give me permission to be rude. Reminding myself that I could not immediately say what came to mind, I knew I would have to apply my filter before opening my mouth in the future. Was I turning into my mom?

Mom remained strangely quiet during the time we were at the hospital. At about 10:30 p.m., another nurse practitioner arrived and informed us that they would be admitting Mom. Once again, we had to review her medical history, medications, and needs. We arranged for meals to be automatically delivered and instructed the staff that she needed assistance with feedings if she ate. They confirmed that things would be done as we requested, and I was grateful.

I sent Meisha a text to let her know Mom had been admitted to Central Hospital and that I wanted her to report to the hospital at noon on Friday and stay there until her shift was over. Our family didn't want to risk losing Meisha, so we agreed that we would pay her full-time wages when Mom was either in the hospital or in the rehab facility. This ensured that she would not feel the need to find fill-in work; we did not want to take the chance that she might find another full-time assignment. Additionally, having her come to the hospital provided us with some peace of mind. Mom would be able to receive the extra attention we felt she needed.

I was comforted knowing someone I trusted would be with her until I returned. I told Meisha to call me if she had questions and let her know that I'd call her once I had more information. At about 11:00 p.m., someone informed us that the hospital was full, and that Mom would remain in the ER until a bed became available in the main hospital. Daniel and I stayed until about 11:30, when Mom was snoring so loudly that we were assured she was resting. We felt she would sleep through the night due to all the medications she had been given.

We were quiet on the ride home. When I asked if he wanted to pick up something to eat, he declined stating there was food at the house. I had brought lunch to Mom's home earlier, which she obviously hadn't eaten, and decided that would be my dinner. I planned to arrive at the hospital early Friday morning with the hopes of speaking with whichever physician would be tending to Mom. Sleep eluded me that night, and I don't believe Daniel slept either.

I arrived at the hospital at about 9:00 a.m. on Friday and learned Mom had been moved from the ER to a regular room. She was sleeping when I reached her room, and I noticed there was no breakfast. Meals were supposed to arrive automatically, so why was there no breakfast in her room? Realizing that I was extremely stressed, I willed myself to take a couple of cleansing breaths: Breathe in through the nose, then slowly release the air through your mouth. I remember saying that phrase countless times during my "Reducing Caregiver Stress" presentations. I needed to practice what I preached.

Mom's breakfast was delivered shortly thereafter, although she wanted nothing to do with it. She surprised me by asking for water, drinking a full cup, and requesting more. Many thoughts ran through my mind. She hadn't eaten at all the previous day but was refusing food. She had to be hungry, or was her body beginning to shut down, no longer requiring food? Had the dementia reached the point where she needed cues to know when or how to eat? Was the *C. diff* curtailing her appetite? There was so much symptom overlap that I couldn't be sure what was going on.

Because her desire for fluids had reappeared, I decided that the *C. diff* had more than likely been the reason for the lack of appetite. I guess I'd officially promoted myself to "physician." I hoped that she would eat more once the *C. diff* was managed.

I went to the nurse's station to let the nurse know that I wanted to speak with Mom's attending physician when he or she became available. Upon reviewing the whiteboard hanging on the wall in her room, I saw that her physician was actually a nurse practitioner and that Mom had been admitted under observation. I chuckled to myself. I didn't care that she was not actually admitted because Daniel and I had agreed that Mom would not be returning to the rehab facility. As such, Medicare's three-day admittance rule (required for Medicare to pay for rehab) was not a concern.

Lesson: For Medicare to cover a person's stay at a SNF, he or she must have a qualifying hospital admittance. As of this writing, a qualifying admittance involves being admitted to the hospital for a minimum of three days/nights. Being admitted under observation does not qualify.

When the nurse practitioner came into Mom's room, he did not volunteer much information. I had learned to be patient when it came to physicians, allowing them to speak before asking questions. Oftentimes, they answered the questions I had before I asked them, but sometimes they didn't. He didn't.

I threw a barrage of questions at him. "What is going on with Mom's pneumonia? Is it a new case or residual from the time before? Why are her creatinine numbers almost three times higher than they had been in February? Could you please explain these blood test results to me because I am having trouble understanding their significance? What are these 'low-density masses' that are at the base of her spine and in her upper abdomen?" He barely got the word "probably" out of his mouth when I interrupted. "Please don't say the word probably to me. I want definitive answers." To say he was taken aback would be an understatement.

He quickly learned that he was not dealing with a passive family member. I wanted answers. "Much of what you are asking is unrelated to this admittance," he said. I snapped, "Don't tell me that this or that has nothing to do with this admittance. I have learned new information that was not available to me before. Since these conditions were not relayed to us during Mom's last admittance, they need to be addressed now." The nurse practitioner stated that he would be ordering CT scans of Mom's lungs, abdomen, and spine, and making a referral to a nephrologist to address my concerns regarding her creatinine levels. I was happy with his plan and thanked him as he hurriedly left Mom's room. I smiled at myself. Objective met.

If you haven't already guessed, I had gained access to Mom's medical records and took the time to review them. Even though Daniel and I had decided to focus on comfort care for Mom, I didn't see how appropriate comfort measures could be implemented if we were unaware of everything that was going on.

> **Lesson:** Most medical records are online these days. Encourage your loved ones to set up an online account so their records can be regularly reviewed. Offer to hold the passwords for them so you will have access, or in case they lose or forget them. If you haven't done so, set up an account for yourself as well.

I was relieved when Meisha arrived at the hospital. She would be able to make sure that Mom received her meals and assist with feeding her if needed. In essence, Meisha would serve as Mom's "call button." I did not expect her to do the work of the hospital staff, but wanted her to ensure the hospital staff were providing Mom with what she needed when she needed it.

I shared with Meisha some of the behaviors I had noticed with Mom. "If she begins to smack her lips together, offer her water. If she kicks her covers off, she either needs to be toileted or changed. When she fidgets with her blanket, she is more than likely agitated," I said. As I prepared to leave, I asked Meisha to call me if anything came up and to let me know how things went during the afternoon. Knowing Daniel would relieve Meisha once his work shift was over, I kissed Mom, told her I loved her and that I would return the following day. She did not respond.

When I reached my car, I just sat for a moment. Suddenly, I found myself trying to remember the last time Mom had followed my saying "I love you" with her usual response, "I love you always." I couldn't recall the last time I'd heard those words and was overcome by sadness. I felt an overwhelming need to call George. I missed him so much. He had been more patient than I could have imagined. He never complained about my time away, only asking me if and how he could be of assistance. He picked up Ann from school and watched her until her Mom got off work. He was so supportive, and I did not take for granted for one moment how blessed I was to have him as my life partner.

I called and his first words were, "How are you doing, dear?" I told him things were rough and that I was very sad. When he asked if there was anything he could do to help, I told him that he'd already done more than I'd expected. I just needed to hear his voice and told him how much I loved him. He told me that he loved me too and asked if I was okay to drive. I told him that I'd be fine and would see him shortly.

As I hung up the phone my tears began to flow, continuing to flow freely throughout my drive home. Whenever I had to stop at a light, I put my head down because I didn't want anyone in a car next to me to see me crying. I don't know why I cared what a stranger would think, but I did.

I was tired and, I admit, depressed. I was depressed! I was holding it together, but not sure how long I could do so. As long as I was busy, I was fine. It was when I stopped moving and had time to think about the reality of what was happening, that I felt like everything would fall apart. The irony of all of this was that for years, I had done presentations about the importance of caregivers taking care of themselves. I knew the steps and the tricks, but again I was learning what the books can't teach. When real life hit, those knowings seemed to go right out of the window. I knew better, but I wasn't doing better. I'd rest . . . later.

I thought about how I had always tried to encourage people to take advantage of the many support services available through the Alzheimer's Association. Again, I was not practicing what I preached. I felt the need to do it all. I didn't have time to try to get assistance and support. That's not true. I had the time but chose to use my time differently. Crazy, right?

George was waiting at the door when I arrived home. He could see our driveway from his recliner and always met me at the door when I arrived home from anywhere. That made me feel as if he'd missed me and was happy I was home. I felt loved! When he opened the door, I just collapsed into his arms and broke down. I released all the emotion that had been bottling up inside.

He just held me, which was exactly what I needed at that moment. He assured me that I was doing all that I possibly could for Mom and that I should feel good about that. He reminded me of how fortunate I was to have the support of my siblings; not all families worked together like mine. He told me that I was lucky my job had provided me with so much valuable knowledge which, in turn, helped me understand what was going on and the important questions that needed to be asked. Even though I didn't know whether that knowledge was a blessing or a curse, I slept better that night.

Lesson: No one is invincible. Depression is not a sign of weakness. Recognition of what's going on is important. Don't be afraid to ask for the help you need.

Later that evening, I used the computer to retrieve the results of Mom's earlier tests. She had so much going on! In addition to everything mentioned previously, the CT scan showed her emphysema was moderate to severe, she had compression fractures and healed rib fracture deformities, and other issues. Initially, I was angry about the fractures, which did not show on the CT scan she had in February. But then I reminded myself that I could not be angry with anyone about the fractures.

Mom was constantly falling, everywhere. She'd fallen at home, while out with friends, at the SNF, and in the hospital. No one could be blamed because not one of us had been able to protect her from falling—and I felt guilty about that. Now was the time for me to move beyond anger and guilt and focus on putting as many safety precautions in place for her as possible.

> **Lesson:** The best you can do is the best you can do.

My brothers and I agreed to meet at Mom's on Saturday to discuss how we would be moving forward. I decided to take that opportunity to discuss hospice care. I had printed pages from Mom's most recent medical records and had collected literature about hospice to share with them. I didn't know if they had preconceived notions about hospice or if they knew anything at all about it. This was going to be an education session. I was going to try to take off my daughter/sister hat and put on my community educator hat. My goal was to share facts while trying to hold my emotions at bay, because we needed consensus on how we would move forward.

I had been involved with Hospice of the Western Reserve for years, first as a volunteer and later as an employee. In my eyes, they were the best, having provided quality end-of-life care for more than thirty-five years, I considered them to be the experts. The training they provided for paid and non-paid staff was exceptional. My former coworkers and fellow care team members were some of the most compassionate and caring individuals I had ever known, seeing their work as a calling as opposed to a job. In my opinion, if we decided to move forward and place Mom under the care of hospice, HWR was my obvious choice.

My brothers were waiting for me when I arrived at Mom's home, and I was ready for business. I passed out copies of Mom's medical records while verbally summarizing what was noted. I let them know that the doctors had asked Daniel and me how aggressive we wanted them to be with Mom's treatment plan, explaining that she had reached a point where she was having a harder time fighting off infections and that the infections would continue to recur. We were basically on a treadmill, putting forth the effort but not going anywhere. We could continue the cycle of Mom getting ill, going to the hospital, and then going to rehab until she died. "Do we think that's what Mom would want?" I asked. Everyone said no.

It was then that I mentioned what the physicians seemed to be hesitant to bring up: hospice care. I couldn't help but notice the look on Don's face when the H-word was mentioned. I asked what he knew about hospice and he said, "I know that everyone who goes on hospice dies." I said, "People don't die because they go under hospice care. They go under hospice care because they are dying." There. I'd finally said it. My mom was dying. "It doesn't mean that she's dying today or tomorrow or next month. The doctor just certifies that if her disease runs its normal course, she will probably die within six months. Persons with dementia sometimes live longer than anticipated. It's speculated that this is the case because they are unaware of their condition and how ill they really are. Curative measures would be stopped, and the focus would be on doing whatever would be needed to keep Mom comfortable."

Lesson: Hospice is the last rung on the ladder of the continuum of care. It is utilized when someone has been given months versus years to live. The focus of hospice is to enhance the overall quality of life for as long as that life lasts. Hospice care does not impede nor accelerate the dying process.

I reminded my brothers of Mom's desire to be at home, even though she lacked awareness of where home actually was. I explained to them that hospice care would allow us to keep her comfortable providing an aide to help with her personal care, like baths, nail care, shampooing, etc. Mom would also be assigned a nurse who would manage her medical needs, with a physician available if needed. Other services would include a social worker and a spiritual care coordinator.

When I asked if they felt hospice should be the direction we should take, everyone nodded yes. When I asked if they felt we should have further discussion or if they had any hesitation, they all responded no. Then came the conversation regarding which hospice provider we should use. Of course, I advocated for HWR. Nicholas, however, stated that the staff at the nursing home where he worked were strong advocates of Crossroads Hospice, speaking extremely highly of them. I was familiar with Crossroads because they were a strong competitor of HWR. To add to the mix, Central Hospital, where Daniel worked, also provided hospice services.

In my opinion, because Central Hospital's hospice was relatively new, I objected to considering them for Mom. I admit that I was biased but also realized that I needed to be open to the idea that another hospice would be capable of providing the quality of care I would expect for my mom. It was decided that Daniel and I would meet with a social worker at Central to see what their experiences had been with Crossroads and HWR. Nicholas and Don trusted us to make the final decision.

Our meeting concluded close to lunchtime, and—you guessed it—I was going to prepare fried green tomatoes for Mom. Since she had a good appetite the previous day, according to Meisha, surely she would be able to enjoy one of her favorite meals today. I arrived at the hospital at 12:40 p.m. Once I reached her floor and entered the hallway, I recognized Mom's cough. I then recognized her voice and thought to myself, "She must be feeling better!" She was fussing and cussing up a storm.

My first thought when I entered her room was, What the hell? Both Mom and her bed were covered in some type of red powder. Glancing sideways, I saw a near-empty bag of Fiery French Fries. Who had given her those? As I began to clean up the mess, she looked up, saw me, and said, "Who the hell are you, and what are you doing in my house?" I bit my lip and told her I was her daughter.

She looked me dead in the eye and said, "Prove it!" I said, "Prove I'm your daughter?" and she said, "Yes." I told her the story of my birth that I'd heard her tell so many times: "You and Dad had four sons already when you found out you were pregnant with me. When I was born, and Dad was told I was a girl, he stripped the diaper off me to see if it was true. He was so excited and proud to be the father of a daughter.

139

He named me LaBena because someone told him it was Spanish for 'my baby,' but they were wrong. Do you believe I'm your daughter now?" She said, "I guess."

As I looked at Mom, it was obvious that she had not been bathed or changed; clean clothing rested on a nearby shelf. I took a calming breath and walked to the nurse's station, where an aide I had previously met was present. I asked if she knew who had given Mom the Fiery French Fries; she had no idea. When I asked why there was no lunch tray in Mom's room, she said she didn't know. I again took a deep breath before speaking further.

I asked the aide if Mom had eaten breakfast, and she said Mom had refused it. I then told her that whether Mom had eaten the previous meal or not, I expected that breakfast, lunch, and dinner would be automatically delivered and that someone would be available to help her eat it. I knew Mom was difficult, but that was no excuse for not offering her food and keeping her clean. I told her that if Mom needed to be medicated to get those things done, so be it.

Lunch was ordered, and the aide, along with a nurse, came to clean Mom and change her bedding. "Dammit. I don't need you to clean me. I can clean my damn self. I can change my bed, too. Get the hell out of my house," she screamed. I said, "Mom, look how dirty you and your bed are. There is red powder from your fries all over the place. You don't want to lie in this mess. Let these nice ladies help you." She reluctantly allowed herself to be cleaned, stating that she would do it herself next time. I smiled and told her that she could certainly do it herself next time, knowing full well that she would not remember what she'd said.

Mom became more agitated, complaining about all the strangers coming into her home. I recommended that she be given something for anxiety but, as was becoming more prevalent, she refused the medication, and Daniel had to be summoned to assist. After a few moments, he was able to encourage her to take her meds. He had the Midas touch as far as being able to garner compliance from Mom.

She refused the tomatoes I had prepared and became irate when I asked her multiple times if she wanted to try them. I believed she didn't know who I was and wasn't about to eat anything she felt a stranger had prepared. The only thing I was able to get her to eat was the small cup of sherbet that was on her lunch tray, and without objection, she allowed me to feed it to her. As I did so, I realized that this was the first time I'd ever fed my mom. In my mind, I could hear her saying, "I need to do whatever I can for myself. If I don't use it, I'll lose it." Had she lost it?

When she asked why so many people were in her house, I broke another dementia rule. I explained she was in the hospital and that people were there to help her. I silently prayed that she wouldn't become more agitated, and she didn't. Thank you, God!

During my time with her, the infectious disease doctor entered the room. She asked Mom what year it was and Mom said, "Twenty-eight." She asked Mom if she knew who I was, and she said, "She is supposed to be my daughter." Ouch! The doctor told me she planned to put Mom on a thirty-day course of vancomycin for her *C. diff*. I was nervous because I knew antibiotic use could cause or intensify the *C. diff*, but was unsure what other options existed. I was too exhausted to ask any further questions.

I was also able to see the nephrologist who was seeing Mom because of her decreased kidney function. She felt some of Mom's kidney issues could have been the result of the blood pressure medications she was on. She planned to discontinue some of those medications, decrease the dosage of others, and monitor the impact. I was pleased with that news as I was having difficulty understanding why she was on so many in the first place.

When I saw that Mom was falling asleep, I decided to leave and try to get some rest myself. I had hoped to speak with her attending physician to discuss our desire for hospice and their plans for discharge, but that didn't happen. As I was leaving, I requested that the nurse please ask the attending physician to call me, although I didn't expect him to.

After calling and updating my brothers, I drove home. Once I arrived, I saw that I'd received a text from my cousin Ronnie informing me that her husband Charles, who was in pharmaceutical sales, had told her that a drug called DIFICID was the gold standard for treating drug-resistant *C. diff.* I decided to discuss that with Mom's doctor to see why it had not been offered as an option for treatment. After filling George in on the happenings of the day, without tears this time, I lay down and took a much-needed, three-hour nap.

When I awakened, I researched DIFICID online. After seeing the lowest GoodRx price at the time ($3,836 for twenty tablets), I knew why that particular drug had not been recommended. Gold standard or not, I knew no one would recommend prescribing such an expensive medication for someone in Mom's condition.

At 10:00 p.m., I received a call from Dr. Green, who was the physician assigned to my mom that day. I was shocked and amazed that he had called me. He stated that he was sorry to be calling so late but that he had worked from noon until nine and wanted to review Mom's records before calling me. He asked what concerns I had, and I said I was trying to get a sense of whether he felt my brothers and I had made the right decision to have Mom placed on hospice care.

Dr. Green stated that he felt that the decision was "very ethical," which I thought was an interesting term to use. He reiterated what we had heard from the ER physicians. We spoke of Mom's age, the infections, and her challenges bouncing back after each new incident. After speaking with him for about twenty minutes, I felt confident in our decision and was grateful that he had called.

Dr. Green said that he would have his colleague, who would be taking over Mom's case, call me on Sunday with further updates. I really couldn't believe the level of service I was receiving and felt immense gratitude. Dr. Green stated that he wished us the best, and we ended our call.

As promised, on Sunday I received a call from Mom's assigned physician, Dr. Jonas. He let me know that she was having a pretty good day and asked if I had any concerns. I shared the same information that I had told Dr. Green. Dr. Jonas was not as definitive in his responses as Dr. Green had been, seeming to be more focused on how she was at that instant as opposed to reviewing her history. I felt that he may not have been totally on board with the idea of hospice; however, he eventually agreed it was the appropriate level of care for Mom.

I let him know how thankful I was for his call and told him I would be coming in on Monday to see Mom. Dr. Jonas felt it would be a good idea to have me speak with their hospice nurse to get her opinion regarding whether Mom was ready for hospice care. I let him know that our family was considering either HWR or Crossroads. He responded that we would still be required to speak with their hospice nurse first and could move forward from there.

Lesson: You have the right to choose which hospice provider you want to care for your loved one. Others may offer suggestions, but the ultimate decision is yours.

I asked if the discharge plan was in place. He told me that the plan would be done once the final decision was made regarding hospice care. If she was not going on hospice, the recommendation would be to return her to rehab. That was not going to happen! I hoped we would be given the time we needed to do whatever needed to be done before Mom was released, and he assured me that such would be the case. When I advised him I would be returning to the hospital around 9:30 a.m. on Monday, he said that he and the hospice nurse would meet me and Daniel in Mom's room. I was surprised, but pleased, by that statement.

I arrived at Mom's room by 9:20 on Monday morning, with Daniel arriving shortly thereafter. Over the course of the next one and a half hours, Daniel left for work and returned multiple times because the doctor and nurse had not arrived as promised. Recognizing that the physician had scheduled the meeting without speaking to the nurse first,

I decided to be patient. We finally had the nurse paged at 11:00. She came to the room, apologized and explained how busy she had been, and asked if we could meet at 11:30. We said yes.

While waiting, my sister-in-law Grace, my nephew Lucas, and two of his children arrived to visit Mom. Grace shared that when Don had visited with Mom on Sunday, she told him that she needed to see her grandchildren so she could go. Now some things made sense to me. Mom had been fixated on her grandchildren since I'd arrived. She would name her children and then recite the names of her grandchildren, in order of their birth. I was fascinated that she was able to do that with one hundred percent accuracy, even though she hadn't recognized any of her visitors.

As promised, the hospice nurse returned at 11:30 and Daniel and I followed her to a conference room. After introductions, we delved right into Mom's medical history. Being a bit anal, I had notes about everything she had been going through for the last six weeks. After all the information was presented to the nurse, and after she reviewed Mom's chart, she agreed that hospice care was appropriate for Mom.

When I asked what she felt the qualifying diagnosis would be, to my surprise she said, "Emphysema." I'm not sure what I expected, but emphysema wasn't on my list. She did say she was not sure what diagnosis would be used, but she was sure Mom was hospice-appropriate. She began to plan for Mom to go under the care of Central's hospice until I objected, stating we were considering two other providers. I told her that Central's hospice was too new and that I wasn't comfortable using them.

She stated that as a Central employee, she was required to at least offer their hospice services, but the final decision was ours. I asked her to please share the experiences she'd had with each of the providers we were considering: Crossroads and HWR. She responded that HWR had an excellent reputation (which I already knew), especially in Cuyahoga County, but that it did not have a strong presence in Portage County because they were fairly new to the area. I could not disagree.

She said that Crossroads had been in Portage County for a long time and had a strong presence. If we were talking about Mom being served in Cuyahoga County, she'd select HWR without hesitation. But for Portage County, she had to go with Crossroads. She felt Mom would require quite a bit of attention and that Crossroads had the level of presence required to meet her needs.

As Mom's health care power of attorney (HCPOA), Daniel felt Crossroads would be a better choice. We anticipated many issues/problems once Mom got home, and responsiveness was important to us. I agreed with Daniel that Crossroads, because of its established presence in Portage County, was the right choice, understanding that we could change providers at any time if we were not satisfied with their service.

Lesson: Your first priority is to advocate for your loved ones. Make decisions based upon their needs, not your loyalties.

I was heading home from the hospital when I received a call from a representative from Crossroads, asking if I could meet at the hospital in two hours. I reluctantly declined, offering to meet the following day instead. She then told me they would need to meet with Mom's HCPOA to get things moving. I told her Daniel was her HCPOA and worked at the hospital, and then provided his phone number.

Daniel met with her that afternoon and signed consent forms to begin hospice care. The plan was that needed supplies would be delivered to Mom's home on Tuesday morning, and Mom would be discharged later in the day. I received a call from the admitting person and arranged to have her transported home after 6:00 p.m. on Tuesday. Sigh! I again expressed gratitude to George for wanting me to retire and to God for showing me the way. I wanted to be actively involved in Mom's care, which would have been extremely difficult if I were still working.

The Lord is my strength and my shield; my heart trusted in Him, and I am helped: therefore my heart greatly rejoiceth; and with my song will I praise Him. Psalms 28:7

Chapter 19
What Now?

Daniel had arranged for equipment to be delivered to Mom's home early Tuesday morning and planned to go to work right afterward. I had an appointment to have my hair done that morning. Because I'd neglected my hair for so long, I felt I deserved to take some time for myself. I shouldn't have felt guilty about it, but I did. When I arrived at Mom's at 11:30, Daniel was still there. He said the delivery had not come early as promised and decided to wait for it, as opposed to having one of the other siblings come over. He didn't want to bother anyone, he said. He then left for work as I waited for the equipment.

Had we been thinking, we could have had Meisha wait at the house for the equipment instead of going to the hospital that morning. Hindsight is twenty-twenty! Once the equipment was delivered, I decided to hang out at the house and do some last-minute prep for Mom's return instead of waiting at the hospital for her transport team. I prepared a small pot of collard greens and some cornbread, knowing she loved both and hoping she'd want to eat later. I also did some last-minute tidying. At 4:30, I decided to go to the hospital to relieve Meisha and wait for the transport company to come.

When Daniel came to Mom's room after he got off work, I suggested he go home and relax a bit. I said, "Both of us don't need to be here for transport." He agreed, so I knew he was tired. While waiting, my nephew, Thomas, arrived with his family. Mom was happy to see them, but I noticed Thomas looked uneasy. This was the first time he'd seen Mom since Lewis' funeral, and he was unnerved by her appearance. He later said that he'd always felt my side of the family was invincible and that it was difficult to see Grandma that way. I found the term "invincible" odd since Mom had buried three sons. Perhaps he meant to say that he thought my mom was invincible.

In a way, I think all of us viewed her as invincible. She had survived a nasty divorce from the love of her life and the death of three of her children. She was a survivor! I kept observing Thomas as he paced in and out of Mom's room and saw the sadness etched in his face. I understood, but I couldn't help him. He had his demons to contend with, and they had to be dealt with in his way. I was carrying my own weight and not strong enough to carry the weight of anyone else. I wasn't being insensitive by not attempting to provide comfort to him. I was merely choosing to put my "oxygen mask" on first.

My focus returned to Mom. Although she knew (and seemingly understood) that she was going home, she was unusually patient and calm. Don't get me wrong; she was more than ready to go. What I found interesting was the fact that she was not angry or agitated while waiting for the transport team to come. When they finally arrived, she was pleasant and joked with them as they wrapped her in a blanket and placed her onto the gurney that would carry her to the waiting van. Even when I left her to go to my car, she didn't protest. She just wanted assurance that I would be home when she got there, and I confirmed that I would be.

Once we arrived at Mom's home and reached her bedroom, she asked for her purse so that she could pay the nice gentlemen who had transported her. We all got a kick out of that! After we had gotten her changed and into bed, Daniel convinced her to take a breathing treatment because she was coughing harshly and constantly. After the treatment, the coughing was not as intense and Mom asked for something to eat, which excited us. She hadn't asked for food in a long time. Was she rallying again?

I went to warm up the food I'd prepared earlier and made a small plate for her. Unfortunately, Mom ate only a few bites before announcing she was full. Yes, I know she had been eating very little, but these were greens! Not only did she not eat much, but she also began to violently cough again. I feared she was going to aspirate.

A hospice nurse arrived two hours later to provide tuck-in service, which consisted of her assessing Mom's condition and recording the information. We then went to the dining room to discuss the next steps. The nurse reviewed medications to see what would be continued, discontinued, or added, answered our questions, and informed us which staff would be a part of the care team that would be arriving within twenty-four hours.

I have to say that I struggled when we were told that her cholesterol, blood pressure, and thyroid medications were all being discontinued. I knew hospice meant comfort care, not cure, but I also knew that hospice was not supposed to hasten death. Discontinuing those medications could hasten death, but in reality, those medications were possibly prolonging her life. Knowing that didn't make acceptance any easier. My heart was again in conflict with my head.

When we were told that the vancomycin Mom was taking for her *C. diff* infection was to be discontinued, I lost it. My argument was that we wanted the patient, my mom, to be comfortable. How could she be comfortable if she was experiencing uncontrolled diarrhea? She couldn't! I was adamant that the vancomycin be continued, and I was going to fight for that. The nurse excused herself so she could call her supervisor to discuss my concern and returned stating that the vancomycin would be continued.

When the nurse went back to Mom's room to complete her assessment, Mom was tired and didn't want to be bothered; however, she reluctantly complied. Her blood pressure was 90/60 and her pulse ox was 88. Obviously, she no longer needed her blood pressure medication, but she certainly needed her oxygen. She was not experiencing any pain and, despite her cough, appeared to be doing well. I was happy she was resting at home instead of in the hospital or at a SNF. She didn't even realize that her big, comfortable bed had been replaced with a hospital bed. Thank goodness!

Six Days until Ninety!

The nurse left, and Daniel and I had a late dinner. We were quiet, thinking and reflecting on the fact that Mom was now facing her final journey. We were sad, and neither one of us wanted to speak about what was going on. I decided to stay overnight because I wanted to be there to meet Mom's hospice care team on Wednesday. We looked in on her, said our goodnights, and went to bed.

Daniel got up multiple times during the night to check on Mom; I jumped up each time I heard him. He did not want any assistance with anything, and I was able to see just how devoted he was to her.

His voice was soft, and his touch was tender. He was patient and kind. The love was so evident. I was a little jealous of the connection I witnessed between them, but the jealousy was short-lived because of the beauty of it all. The son was caring for the mother who had once cared for him. The son was caring for the mother who had made the past few years a living hell. The son was caring for the mother because he truly loved her and treasured her.

My heart broke as I thought of how her passing would impact Daniel. I was beginning to understand why my mom had once asked me if Daniel would be okay. I now saw the reason for her concern; I was becoming concerned as well. Daniel always seemed so calm, cool, and collected, rarely showing his emotions. What would it take to get him to release?

Five Days until Ninety!

The nurse assigned to Mom's care was named Jenna, and she was an angel. When she came to the house Wednesday morning, compassion exuded from her. She took the time to explain all services, confirm who Mom's other care providers would be, and answer any questions I had. She also answered Meisha's questions, since she would be the one who would be with Mom most days.

In many ways, fifteen-plus years of being involved with HWR had prepared me for what to expect with my mom, but in other ways, I was totally unprepared. I had very good knowledge of the services that would be provided and knew how things were supposed to work. If I knew so much, why couldn't I remember anything? As Jenna spoke, I felt as though I were hearing and learning everything for the first time.

I asked what they were using as Mom's terminal diagnosis and was surprised when Jenna said late-stage Alzheimer's disease. I had been so focused on all the other symptoms and illnesses Mom had that it had totally escaped me that she was experiencing signs of end-stage Alzheimer's. As I reflected back, it was obvious.

According to the Alzheimer's Association, when someone is in the latter stages of Alzheimer's disease, they may experience the following:

- Need round-the-clock assistance with daily activities and personal care
- Lose awareness of recent experiences as well as of their surroundings
- Experience changes in physical abilities, including the ability to walk, sit, and, eventually, swallow
- Have increasing difficulty communicating
- Become vulnerable to infections, especially pneumonia

Although we had been seeing evidence of all of these, their manifestations had been overshadowed by the severity of the symptoms she was experiencing due to her many infections. The onset of those infections had more than likely been the result of her diminished immunity because of Alzheimer's.

I recalled teasing Daniel that the only time I saw Mom smile was when she would smile at him. It never occurred to me that she could be losing her ability to smile. Surprisingly, in the past few days, Mom had been smiling more, oftentimes while looking up to a corner in the room. When I'd ask her what she was smiling at, she would say, "Nothing." It was as if she had a secret that she was not going to share.

This person, who thought she had known so much, had missed the signs that her mother was dying from dementia. Everything else would just be considered a co-morbidity (contributing factor). Who knew?

Jenna asked me to share the things I had noticed going on with Mom. Because I kept extensive notes, I was able to recount pretty much everything: three hospitalizations in less than two months, pneumonia (three times); *C. diff* (two times); VRE sepsis; UTI (two times); sleeping more; minimal intake of food and fluids; unstable blood pressure and pulse ox; lethargy; garbled/nonsensical speech (intermittent); bed-bound; leg and back pain; agitation and combativeness; depression; and heavy cough. I had barely gotten the word *cough* out of my mouth when I began to sob uncontrollably.

Speaking aloud all that my poor mom had been going through these past several weeks broke my heart. I tried to compose myself because I didn't want Mom to hear me, but I couldn't control my emotions. Jenna got up from her chair, placed her arms around me, and told me to let it out. I noticed tears rolling down Meisha's cheeks as well. It was then that I stopped crying. This was not the time for me to fall apart, I thought. I had to put my big girl panties on and be about my mother's business, at least for now.

After Jenna completed her interview with me, it was time for her to meet and examine my mom. Earlier, Mom had asked if she was going to the doctor today. I wondered if that was her way of telling me she didn't feel well and told her the doctor would be coming to see her. When we reached her room, I let her know the "doctor" was there to see how she was doing. Surprisingly, she was cooperative as Jenna examined her.

Mom's blood pressure and pulse ox were low again. Her breathing was shallow, and she was lethargic. She didn't seem to have any fight left in her. I looked at Jenna's face and saw a deep sadness in her eyes. I knew she'd probably witnessed many deaths, and I was touched by the compassion that seemed to exude from her. As I watched her tenderness with Mom, I was comforted.

We went back to Mom's dining room table, the family gathering place, and Jenna jotted down a few notes. I asked her point-blank how long she thought we were looking at. "Maybe a week or two," she said. But in my heart of hearts I didn't feel Mom would make it beyond the weekend. Hearing she might make it a week or two should have given me some hope, but I didn't believe it.

I let Jenna know that we all believed that Mom was holding on for her ninetieth birthday, which was five days away. I didn't think she'd live to see it but had been praying that God would allow it. I know prayers aren't always answered with "yes," but that didn't stop me from asking. Miracles happen every day. Right?

Jenna then gave me a refresher course on the signs that would be visible as Mom drew closer to death. Those signs included: discoloration and/or mottling (blotchy coloring) of lower extremities; shallow and/or rapid breathing; mouth slacked open to the side; cold feet and/or legs; gurgling . . . the list went on, but I had stopped listening. Although Mom was not exhibiting any of those signs right then, in the recent past I had witnessed everything Jenna had mentioned, except the mottling and gurgling.

I asked Jenna how long she thought it would be once we saw those signs, and she said, "Usually within a week." That would be about right, I thought to myself. Jenna then said Mom's team would consist of an aide, a nurse, a social worker, a chaplain, and a physician. Her records showed Mom's primary care physician had chosen to continue to care for her throughout her hospice journey, and I was happy about that. He had a personal connection with Mom, and I knew he would stay on top of things.

Jenna reminded me of the number we should call if there was anything we needed, and that hospice was available 24/7. She said that support would increase if and when we thought Mom was actively dying, reiterating that our family was not in this alone. She gave me a big hug and told me the social worker would be contacting me soon.

153

Before Jenna's vehicle had left the driveway, I received a call from Jane, the social worker, asking if she could come by to meet Mom. She arrived within the hour. We made small talk, and I discovered that HWR had cared for both of her parents when they were dying before she joined the staff at Crossroads. How ironic was that?

I took her up to meet Mom, who was initially unaware of her presence. Jane asked for permission to come to see her occasionally, and Mom said, "That would be fine." When Jane and I returned to the table, she asked if I could answer some questions for her. She then interviewed me about my mom's upbringing, work history, children, grandchildren, great- and great-great grandchildren, hobbies, and likes/dislikes. She reviewed their services and reminded me that they'd be available 24/7.

I mentioned the fact that Mom was devoutly Catholic but had been unable to attend church in a long time. She asked if I thought Mom would like for a priest to visit. I responded, "Priest, or one of your chaplains?" She said, "Priest." I told her Mom would love that if she was aware of what was going on.

Jane made a few calls and let me know that the pastor of Mom's church had agreed to come to see her on Thursday. Mom's hospice aide, Linda, was also scheduled to come by on Thursday for an introduction. I wondered how Mom would do with so many people coming (the nurse was scheduled to come back as well) and decided I'd better come by again and check on her.

As her visit came to a close, Jane asked me how I was doing and asked whether there was anything I needed. I told her I was doing as well as could be expected but that we were all keeping close watch over Daniel. He appeared to be finding comfort in the care he was providing for Mom, but my other siblings and I were afraid he might be holding his emotions in. Because he was so private, we didn't feel she could be of assistance to him at that time.

As I was doing a mental recap of Jane's visit, I found myself thinking that she had been writing an outline for Mom's obituary. In reality, she was gathering information to help her know Mom better, but it was her obituary. I should know because I'd already written it!

Four Days until Ninety!

At about nine thirty Thursday morning, Meisha called to tell me she was having a difficult time with Mom. She said that Daniel had had difficulty with her as well before he went to work. Mom was refusing her medications and would not get dressed. She had stripped down to nothing during the night and refused to let anyone put clothing on her. The latter was very unusual for her, and Meisha was concerned because she didn't know how Mom would act when her aide and the priest arrived.

Meisha put me on the phone with Mom and that day, I was able to convince her to take her medications. I had especially wanted her to take the antianxiety medication, knowing this would help her get through her visits. I had planned to be there at noon but decided to move my timeframe up with the hopes of ensuring all would go well. Meisha then advised me that Mom's best friend, Barbara, had wanted to come by later but told her that she would need to discuss it with me first. I said I would call Barbara after I'd had an opportunity to see Mom and determine whether she'd be up to a visit. George decided to come with me that day because I had broken the blinds in Mom's bedroom the night before —don't ask—and he needed to replace them. I was curious to see how my mom would react to George since lately she thought I was still married to my first husband, James. He and I had been high school sweethearts, but our marriage was short-lived. How ironic that she would remember him as we had been divorced for more than forty years. Then again, she had dementia and was regressing. Of course, she would remember him.

When we arrived at Mom's home, we learned that Reverend Pierce had just left. Meisha said that the visit had gone well, and that Mom was calm and seemed to recognize Reverend Pierce. It was peculiar that she was alternating between being in and out of confusion. Sometimes she would be oriented times two, and other times she would be oriented times one.

> **Lesson:** The term *oriented* refers to a person's state of awareness and includes self, place, time, and situation. Oriented times one means that a person recognizes him/herself and knows their name but lacks awareness of the other things noted.

When George and I entered Mom's room, she looked up and said, "Hi, George!" That brought tears to my eyes. I had warned George that she might not recognize him because she thought I was still married to James, and we were both pleasantly surprised when she did. She smiled when she said his name.

I told her I had broken her window blinds and asked if it was okay for George to replace them. She said it was okay but that they were just blinds and we didn't need to worry about them. I told her that I had broken them and needed to get them fixed. She smiled and nodded.

Because she seemed alert (although she did not remember that Reverend Pierce had visited), I asked if she would like Barbara to come by. She said, "Of course!" Barbara was extremely happy when I called to let her know it was okay for her to visit. I told her that she would need to gown-up because of Mom's still-active infections. She asked if two o'clock would be a good time to visit; I said that if she wanted Mom to be alert, she might want to come sooner. She agreed.

Meisha let me know that the aide had come by to introduce herself to Mom as well. I was amazed to see that Mom was as alert and cordial as she was in light of all the morning's activities. As was Mom's norm, she looked like she was bouncing back yet again. This was another repeat of her pattern of appearing at death's door one minute and having a miraculous recovery the next.

Barbara arrived with her son Stuart, who drove her, about half an hour after I'd spoken with her. She suited up and went to Mom's bedside. She attempted to make small talk, but she and Mom mostly just looked into each other's eyes and smiled. Barbara spoke of their friendship and Mom occasionally added a word or two. Before Barbara left, she said, "Lottie, you've been a good friend, and I love you." Mom replied, "I love you always." What? That was what she said to me. I had never heard her say that to anyone else, and I wanted it back. That was our thing! I had to rein myself in and look at the beauty of this friendship. I had to accept the fact that I was not the only one my mom would love always.

Mom and Barbara had worked together for many years at the General Electric Company. There was a group of ladies who had retired close to the same time. Since retirement, they would meet for church once a week and go to breakfast afterward. When Mom was no longer able to drive, her friends, Barbara and Eunice, would come by to get her so she wouldn't miss that time with her friends.

During the past several weeks, Barbara and Eunice had been diligent in visiting Mom, exemplifying what true friends should be. I was noticing the toll Mom's experiences were having on Barbara. She seemed to have aged significantly during that short time, moving slower and not standing as tall. There was a deep sadness in her eyes.

How difficult it must be to watch someone so dear to you die. You reach a certain age and that seems to be what you had to look forward to: another death. Mom used to always say, "Just wait till you get old. You'll see what it's like." I wasn't looking forward to that!

Once, when I was on a cleaning frenzy at Mom's (which had become a stress reliever for me), I came across a familiar photograph that my husband had taken many years earlier. Because of all the loss our elders had been experiencing, George and I had decided to host a yearly senior picnic. We wanted our beloved elders to have an opportunity to get together for a joyous occasion, instead of for funerals, so this picnic was held in their honor. We had a huge spread of food, yard and board games, adult beverages, and we would spoil them rotten for the day. We would then take a group photo, which we'd later present to each of them as a memento.

One year, we noticed that the picnic began with the seniors looking at the prior year's photo and pointing out who was now missing. They would then go through the motions of enjoying themselves, but the picnic would have a dark shadow hovering over it. For that reason, we decided to no longer host the event.

As I looked at the photo, I realized that my mom and father-in-law, Benjamin, were the only two originals remaining. Mom was nearing ninety and Benjamin was nearing ninety-four. Benjamin was still in good health and remained active. It wasn't until recently that he'd experienced any health issues. I became sad as I peered at that photo through their eyes.

What was even sadder was the realization that my husband and I were now at the age our seniors had been when that photo had been taken. Although I was still blessed with all my friends, George was seeing the death and decline of many of his.

After ensuring that Mom was comfortable, and seeing she was in a good state of mind, George and I decided to go home. I intended to return on Friday so I would be there for Jenna's follow-up visit. On the way home I didn't feel much like talking, and George respected that. It was a long, silent ride home.

Three Days until Ninety!

Like clockwork, I received a call from Meisha on Friday morning. Mom was raging, had refused her meds from both Daniel and Meisha, and had refused to get dressed. While on the phone, I heard her yell, "Get the hell out of my house," as Meisha attempted to place the phone to her ear so I could try to calm her down. Because I couldn't get to Ravenna before 1:30 p.m. that day, I told Meisha I would call Don to see if he could come by and attempt to calm Mom down. I called and he went right over. He was able to get her to take her meds after several attempts and sat with her until she was calm and resting.

When I arrived, although calm, Mom kept gazing upwards. As I drew closer, I noticed she was calling the names of different deceased people. This wasn't new for Mom. Throughout the past couple of weeks, she would randomly speak of seeing someone who had died. Initially, we thought that her not remembering they were dead was due to her dementia; however, this seemed different.

She would say, "Biney's coming" multiple times. Then she would say this person or that person was coming. I started making note of the names because I didn't recognize many of them. Besides Biney, there was Lucky and Mary Lou, and Dank, whose name she would call incessantly.

At one point, I called Mom's cousin, Nina, who had been raised by Mom's parents, to ask if she knew who these people were. She informed me they were all cousins Mom had grown up with and that they were all deceased. Recalling my hospice training, I thought about visioning. Visioning is when people who are nearing death begin seeing loved ones who have passed before them, as if they are being welcomed to another place. It is a phenomenon that has been witnessed and documented extensively by hospice workers.

I believed Mom was visioning. She mentioned seeing my dad, John III, her dad, and numerous cousins. But there were some I had been expecting her to see that she had not seen yet. She had made no mention of Andrew, Lewis, her mom, or her sister, Nettie. I thought that once she saw them, she would be ready to go.

Jenna arrived, and we sat to discuss the changes we'd seen in Mom. I told her I had been sure Mom wouldn't see her birthday, but she had rallied once again. I said that she had sat up and eaten last night, for Daniel, and that she had been alert that day as well. Jenna looked at me and said, "You never know." I wondered why she was looking at me the way she did. Was that pity I was seeing in her eyes? Then she checked Mom's vitals. Her blood pressure was in the normal range, and her oxygen levels were excellent.

I guess she showed you, I thought. You were looking at me with pity, probably thinking I could not accept the inevitable. You don't know my Lottie, I thought. Then I remembered:

> **Lesson:** Oftentimes, people who are dying will have a sudden burst of energy and awareness a few days prior to death, and then crash.

Was that what we were seeing? When Jenna began reminding me of the signs of someone actively dying, I was confident that she thought Mom's time was shorter than she'd initially anticipated. She first reviewed the Comfort Kit with me. This kit was to be used as needed near the end of life. It included medications for anxiety, pain, fever, and cough . . . just everything you'd need to make someone comfortable, including morphine. She explained how, when, and why each medication was to be used. Although the instructions were on the package, I felt more comfortable after Jenna took the time to explain everything to me.

Then Jenna reminded me of Crossroads' Even More program, where someone would be with us 24/7 during Mom's transition. It was then that I was confident Jenna thought Mom's time was short. I told her the program might be a little overwhelming, but we would be sure to call if we needed them. I thanked her again and saw her to the door.

After a couple of hours, Mom asked if we were going to church. I decided to join her in her thinking and told her we could go on Saturday if she wanted to. She corrected me, stating that you go to church on Sunday, not Saturday. I told her she was absolutely right and wondered if she had reverted to her childhood days as a Baptist, attending services on Sunday. I told her that it would be my honor to join her. She smiled and said, "Alright, we are going to church on Sunday."

I let Meisha leave early, saying that I would stay with Mom until Daniel got home from work. When Daniel arrived, and I was sure that he didn't need me to do anything (Nicholas was scheduled to sit with

Mom while Don took Daniel grocery shopping), I decided to return to my home.

I went back into Mom's room to tell her I'd see her on Sunday, and she asked again if I would go to church with her. I told her that I absolutely would love to go to church with her the next time she went. When I told her I loved her, she replied, "I love you always." That made my heart smile.

I was surprisingly calm during my ride home. I found myself thinking about how I could create "church" for Mom on Sunday. Although her ninetieth birthday would be on Monday, Nicholas and Daniel had to work that day, so we decided to celebrate on Sunday. There were specific people she had been asking for and about, so they were notified of the planned celebration as well. We weren't planning to have all her grandkids come because of the feeling that she would be overwhelmed. Perhaps I could do a small service before the celebration. I just needed to think about what my sermon would focus on; maybe I'd just speak about love and forgiveness, citing a few key scriptures.

Sunday would be Easter Sunday. That's it! I decided I'd use John 3:16 as the focus of my sermon.

For God so loved the world that He gave His only begotten son, so that whosoever believeth in Him should not perish, but have everlasting life. John 3:16

Six weeks ago, I was not sure what type of relationship Mom had with God. This lack of assurance had been a cause of great concern for me. I was a strong believer, and the idea that my Mom might not be deeply troubled me. Such was no longer the case. Mom had called upon God numerous times of late. She was oftentimes seen praying, which I had not seen or heard her do since the last time I had attended a Catholic service with her more than fifty years ago. Isn't that a shame? It comforted me to witness her faith in action. "Thy will be done," I said under my breath.

Then he called for a light, and sprang in, and came trembling, and fell down before Paul and Silas, And brought them out, and said, Sirs, what must I do to be saved? And they said, Believe on the Lord Jesus Christ, and thou shalt be saved, and thy house. Acts 16:29–31

Mom believed in Jesus Christ, recognizing Him as the Son of God who died for our sins. She called out to Him incessantly in the days to come.

Driving home, I received a call from my nephew, Thomas. He was upset because his dad had told him that Mom might not last the weekend. I shared with him that none of us knew when Mom would die. I reminded him of the many times we had thought she was at death's door only to see her make a startling recovery. However, I did share that I felt her time with us would be short. I had been concerned about the time of Mom's death when I was worried about her soul, but I no longer had that worry. I let Thomas know that I did not want to lose my mother, but I also hated that her quality of life was so poor. It would be selfish of us to try to keep her here when she was in such a frail state. He agreed that Mom certainly wouldn't want to continue in her current state.

I told him the names of all the dead visitors to whom Mom had been speaking over the last few days, and how she seemed to have been comforted by them. I told him that I was happy that they were coming to help her transition, which I truly believed was the case.

We spoke of how she lacked awareness of her age and date of birth. Despite that, her prior goal—reaching her ninetieth birthday—had become our goal. We were hoping and praying that this one last wish, although not remembered, could be granted. When I last asked Mom how old she was, she replied, "Three." Ninety meant nothing to her anymore, but it meant everything to us.

I let him know that my siblings and I would be having cake and ice cream for Mom on Sunday in celebration of her upcoming birthday. He shared that Don was scheduled to be with his kids and grandkids (which he hadn't told me) but that he'd make sure Don was at Mom's by two o'clock, our scheduled meeting time.

We spoke more on a variety of topics, and I could sense the relief in my nephew's voice. He seemed to feel better, and so did I.

Two Days until Ninety!
On Saturday, according to Daniel, Mom slept all day.

One Day until Ninety!
The classic car wall clock ticked relentlessly as I finally dragged myself out of bed to prepare for church. I did so with much dread. I wanted Mom to live to see ninety to the point that it had become my obsession, but I just didn't have the confidence that she would. If I had my way, I would have slept through April 1, but that was not an option. I had things to do. Please, not today, Lord!

Today was Resurrection Day, the anniversary of Christ rising from the dead, Easter Sunday. As we prepared for church, I grabbed my phone and turned it on. Normally I would make sure my phone was off during church services, but not today. I found myself thinking that I wanted to be one hundred percent available in case Daniel called to tell me . . . you know! I kept my phone on vibrate and would leave the sanctuary if it went off so I could answer it. I just needed to be available.

During the service, I was engaged some of the time, but at other times I was far removed. I went through the motions but wasn't feeling it. I had greeted fellow attendees and sang the songs, but not really. I received communion and toyed with the idea of taking extra so I could give it to Mom (I didn't). I just wanted this service to end. My mind and heart were elsewhere. I was present, but not really.

I suddenly realized that not only had I forgotten to perform my only assigned task, to buy a "90" candle, but I'd also forgotten to put together

163

an Easter basket for Ann. I had made an Easter basket for her every year since she'd been born. She would never forgive me for forgetting, and I certainly didn't want to disappoint her.

I was grateful we had gone to early service because I had time to go shop for the candle and the fixings for Ann's basket. I became anxious waiting to be dismissed from church and couldn't understand why the service was taking so long. Finally, we were dismissed. May God forgive me for being so distracted and disinterested on His special day, I thought. I was sure He understood.

After first stopping at CVS, I was disappointed to discover they did not have my "90" candle. Adding to my disappointment, my go-to store, Marc's, was closed for the holiday. Luckily, Giant Eagle was not only open but also had my candle. The nearby dollar store had a great selection of cards, treats, and baskets that I could use to put together my gift for Ann. Mission accomplished!

Once I had put the Easter basket together, George and I headed to Ravenna. Mom had been asking for Ann and Lynn, so they would be stopping by. She had also been asking for my stepdaughter Yvonne, and my niece Veda, who both planned to stop by as well. When George and I arrived at 1:30 p.m., Don and Veda were already there. Nicholas then arrived, stating one of his daughters had stopped by earlier.

Because Mom still had *C. diff*, we needed to put on gowns and gloves before entering her room. Daniel suggested that we cut a portion of the cake, put the candle on it, and take only that piece into the room so as not to contaminate the rest of the cake. Why hadn't I thought of that? As we entered the room, Nicholas reminded us to cut off the oxygen before we lit the candle. Mom was glad to have that done and complained that the tubing was uncomfortable.

Lynn, Ann, and my son-in-law Bill arrived just as we began to sing. As we sang "Happy Birthday," Ann blew out the candle for Mom. When Nicholas asked Mom how old she was, she said, "Twenty-eight." She obviously knew she had a connection to the number twenty-eight, the year of her birth, but had no idea what that connection was. I chuckled as I thought of how much she'd aged since Friday when she'd told me she was three. Her age continued to change throughout the time we were with her.

When Yvonne arrived, Mom said she was eighteen. I asked if anything special would happen now that she was eighteen, and she said, "Yes, I can drink!" I found that funny as I knew my mom had begun drinking long before the age of eighteen. She spoke of how much fun she'd had smoking her father's cigars and cigarettes as well. She'd had a good 'ole time!

When we initially arrived, Mom had been somewhat lethargic. Now she was more alert, although confused. She continued to speak of—and to—those who were deceased. She briefly mentioned Biney, but spoke more of her cousin, Dank. She said, "He was a real good kid. He was supposed to wait for me before he went to the wagon, but he didn't. He fell off and he got hurt . . . *real* bad."

Later, she began saying she needed to see the doctor. I asked if she was in pain, and she said she wasn't. When I asked why she needed to see the doctor, she said she needed to get her change. She said that she had "paid him all that money and he didn't do shit!" She then spoke of her former neurologist, Dr. Kincaid. She referred to him as her doctor friend and said that she wanted to go see him. I told her that he didn't work on Sundays but that we would call him on Monday if she'd like. There was no mention of going to church.

Lesson: It is very important to be flexible with your planning. Follow your loved one's lead and recognize that plans may need to be changed based upon how they are feeling and behaving.

Mom ate just a spoonful of cake and about a quarter cup of butter pecan ice cream, her favorite. Then she began talking about buying and cooking collard greens and cornbread. When I let her know that I had already cooked greens and cornbread for her, she asked me to bring some to her. By the time I heated the food and returned to her room, she no longer wanted it. This went on for most of our time with her. She'd ask for something but by the time we'd bring it to her, she either had forgotten she'd asked for it or no longer wanted it.

When she saw Lynn and I told her who she was, she said, "Oh, you're a big girl now." She still remembered Lynn as the little girl who had spent so much time with her and asked for her frequently throughout our visit. She thought Yvonne was my best friend, Lena, just as she had the last time she'd seen her. She initially said that she had never seen George before in her life, but later remembered and asked for him. Seeing Ann and Lynn at the same time was confusing to her: it was as if she were seeing little Lynn and grown-up Lynn simultaneously. Admittedly, Ann looked very much like her mom when she was her age.

Although Mom remained pleasant, you couldn't help but notice how lethargic and tired she was becoming. I was touched when Lynn, who initially had been concerned about exposure to *C. diff*, bent over to hug and kiss her, which was a no-no. It was as if she were saying she didn't care what Mom had; she needed to give her a proper goodbye. We all went one by one to say goodbye, and I told her that I'd see her on Monday. When Bill reached his car, he decided to go back one last time to see Mom. When he returned, he was laughing. He told us that when he'd gone to Mom's room, she asked him who he was. After he explained and said he had been there to wish her a happy birthday, she said, "Well, I guess you've been here long enough."

Mom was resting peacefully when we left her. I didn't get "the call" while at church. She didn't slip away after we sang to her. Perhaps my feelings that she would not live to see her ninetieth birthday were just that, my feelings, and had nothing to do with a message from God. Perhaps all of the friends and family who had been praying for her to see ninety would have their prayers answered. Whatever the case may be, we'd had a nice conversation over her lunch of butter pecan ice cream. She was pain-free. She was at peace. God's will be done.

But seek ye first the kingdom of God, and His righteousness, and all these things shall be added unto you. Matthew 6:33

Chapter 20
Ninety

I don't recall anything about the remainder of that day. I don't remember giving Ann her Easter basket or her reaction to it. I don't recall giving Bill his birthday card (he and Mom shared birthdays), but I know I did. However, I do remember getting a call from Daniel later advising me that Mom had really perked up after everyone had left. That was just like Mom!

I went to bed early, hoping that I'd be able to go to sleep quickly but knowing that I wouldn't. I kept looking at the clock as the minutes and seconds ticked away. Then it happened. It was midnight on April 2, 2018. Mom was officially ninety. For a moment, I wondered if she had died and Daniel chose not to call us because he wanted us to believe she had lived to see ninety. No, he wouldn't do that. Or would he?

I grabbed my phone and sent texts to my brothers saying, "She made it!" I wanted to call but didn't think they were being as anal as I was about everything. I thanked and praised God for allowing Mom to live to see her ninetieth birthday. Although she may not have consciously been aware, I felt that on some level she was. Maybe the prayers and petitions from friends and family requesting that she see this day were answered with a resounding, YES! Perhaps. Whatever the reason, I felt nothing but immense gratitude. The doctors didn't believe she'd make it. The hospice staff didn't believe she'd make it. I didn't think she'd make it, but God said yes. Thank you, Jesus!

Because Meisha would not be available on Tuesday, I planned to arrive at Mom's around three on Monday and stay overnight so I could be with her throughout the following day. I had left instructions for the hospice aide with Meisha, requesting that Mom be given a thorough bed bath, her nails cleaned and clipped, and her hair washed. As I was on my way, Meisha called and said Mom was refusing care. Mom had said, "You ugly bitch. Get the hell out of my house." Why was I not

168

surprised? I had them put the phone to Mom's ear as I tried to convince her to allow them to care for her. Her response was, "No. No. Hell no!" Well, that was that.

By the time I arrived, Jenna was there. She had checked Mom's vitals and said everything, except her breathing, was normal. Mom was sitting on the edge of the bed where I was told she had been most of the day. When I asked if she was tired, she said she was, and she was more than willing to lie down when I suggested she do so. After we got her settled, I walked Jenna to the door. She educated me on the fact that Mom was showing signs that death was close and that she was experiencing a surge of energy that was common when people neared death. She also felt Mom was experiencing *terminal restlessness*. This was another hospice term I was familiar with that was used when patients were experiencing emotional/physical/spiritual anguish, restlessness, anxiety, and agitation. Translation: The time was near.

When I returned to Mom's room and told her to rest, she asked, "Is that woman coming back?" I knew she was referring to Meisha and told her that she would not be back for a couple of days. Mom said, "Good." That made me laugh. I felt Meisha had been doing a great job. Mom just didn't want to be around anyone other than her family. We knew Mom would be resistant to any type of care. Meisha had been charged with keeping Mom clean, safe, and fed—if she would allow it—and Meisha had been doing exactly that. Mom didn't understand that she needed help and did not want to be bothered by "those people."

When Mom fell asleep, I told Meisha she could leave for the day. Shortly thereafter, my best friend Lena came by. She had brought Mom a beautiful floral arrangement and two of her favorite candy bars, Baby Ruth. When Mom awakened, I told her someone was there to see her, and Lena entered the room. Mom looked up at her, smiled, and said, "Lena." Lena presented her with her gifts and asked her how it felt to be ninety. Mom replied, "I don't know." Then, in a childlike voice, she asked, "Will you sing 'Happy Birthday to You'?" Lena replied, "Of course."

As we began to sing, I fell apart. I was completely caught off guard by my reaction and could not continue singing as I listened to Lena finish the song. When she finished singing, Mom said, "You two be best friends forever." In my heart, I believe she was asking my friend to take care of me. Lena told her that we'd been friends for more than fifty years and assured her that we would be friends for the rest of our lives. Mom smiled.

I took a picture of Mom with my phone, then Lena and I each posed with her for more photos. It was a beautiful moment, and I was so grateful to have been able to share it with my best friend. A short time later, Mom drifted off to sleep. Lena and I sat and talked until Daniel came home from work. Nicholas had also decided to stop by to wish Mom a *real* happy birthday.

As Mom slept, we sat and told stories of the fights our parents used to have, laughing as we reminisced. The truth was, we could laugh now but those fights were terrifying at the time. Our parents were the epitome of the saying, "Can't live with them, can't live without them." Telling stories and laughing was our way of coping.

Lena and Nicholas left when Mom was resting and not up to visiting. She did not eat that day, nor was she having any elimination. Her cough became more persistent, so I gave her one of the medications from the Comfort Care kit to assist with mucous and coughing.

That evening, she continued to call out to people who had passed on. It was a little different than it had been in the past. She was more urgent with her calls, not only saying names but also saying, "Show me how." She didn't seem to be distressed; however, per an instruction from Jenna, we gave her antianxiety medication to help settle her down. After a while, she stopped calling and went to sleep. She slept through the night.

The following morning, I heard Daniel get up, so I got up as well. I had been awake for a couple of hours, checking in on Mom periodically and had heard him doing the same. I let him know that if she was hungry when she awakened, I would fix breakfast for her. I told him to just let her sleep, and that I would take care of any personal needs she might have. He allowed me to do that, which surprised me. Although he never asked for help, I knew he appreciated it.

When it was time for her medications, I took them to her. First, I gave her the antibiotic she was still taking for *C. diff* and followed with something to help dry up the mucous that had been accumulating. Although she willingly took both, she spit them out within a few seconds. She had never done that with me before, so I was stunned. After about twenty minutes, I tried to give them to her again, and thankfully, this time she swallowed them. I don't know what changed, but I was grateful for her compliance.

Lesson: If you can't get the desired behavior with your first attempt, walk away and try again later.

She was not hungry, so I left her alone so she could rest. After a brief time, I heard her speaking. As I drew closer, I realized she was praying the Lord's Prayer. I joined her when I noticed she was struggling to remember the words. Then she began calling out to her cousin Dank again. She had been calling and speaking to him so much these last few days. He must have been very special to her. It was odd to think that I had never heard her mention him at all while I was growing up. She was again asking him to show her how. Then she called Biney, asking him to help. She said, "I'm ready to go."

Knowing that many persons with dementia find comfort in listening to music, I had my phone play some of her favorite hymns and left the room. I wanted to let my siblings know that Mom had said she was ready to go. When I returned to her room, Mahalia Jackson was singing "Just a Closer Walk." Mom looked up and said, "Net. You singing?" I said, "Yes, Lot. I am singing some of your favorite songs." I realized that in that moment, Mom thought I was her sister Nettie. She looked over at

171

the wall and smiled. When I asked what she was looking at, she said, "I see Lewis." I asked what he was doing, and she said, "He's smiling."

Before Mom had gone to sleep the night before, she had asked for—or about—several people. She wanted to know how Lynn and Veda were doing. She also asked for her friends Barbara and Eunice, her niece Shawn, and her cousins Nina, Mary, and Stuart. I was surprised she asked for Stuart. Although she had frequently referred to him as one of her favorite cousins, she had been estranged from him for the past several months.

Because of her dementia, she was having many delusions. She called Stuart daily and accused him of stealing all of the inheritance her father had left. I tried to convince her that such was not the case (there was no inheritance to steal), as opposed to redirecting her as I would normally attempt to do. I hadn't spoken with Stuart, but I know how close he and Mom had always been. I was sure he was deeply troubled, not only because Mom thought he would steal from her, but also because Mom treated him so badly.

Despite what I was feeling, I reached out to everyone Mom had mentioned the night before. I called Barbara and Eunice to tell them that she wanted to see them. True to their word, they arrived quickly and within minutes of each other. I left them alone with Mom to say what I thought would be their final goodbyes. They were both tearful as they were leaving. I knew it had to be difficult for them to see their friend withering away, and I wondered if it was easier when someone just died suddenly. Having experienced both, I didn't think either was easier, just different.

Although I wouldn't have traded the time I spent with my mom for anything, the pain of seeing her suffer was, at times, more than I could bear. This time, though, had allowed me and my siblings to grow closer together as we cared for our mom. Each of us did what was needed of us to ensure that we were meeting her needs. By the same token, I believe this was the hardest experience of our lives. Although physically and emotionally draining and depressing, there was some good coming from this experience. God allows things for a reason, even though we may not understand it while we are going through it.

After Barb and Eunice left, I called Mom's niece and her cousins. Mom let Shawn and Mary know how much she loved and wanted to see them. I called Nina and held the phone to Mom's ear. They spoke for a couple minutes, and I could tell it was good for both of them. They were able to tell each other that they loved each other and say their goodbyes. I then called Stuart.

I first spoke to him about Mom's illness and brought him up to date with what she'd been going through. I also assured him of Mom's love for him and that he had always been one of her two favorite people in the whole world before dementia had ravaged her brain. I let him know that she'd asked me to call him for her and asked if he would speak with her. He quickly said he would.

After Mom asked him how he and his family were doing, she told him that she hoped to see him soon. I was hoping they would say they loved each other, but that didn't happen. At least they spoke . . . praise God. I told Stuart that I felt the call had been Mom's way of telling him that she loved him, and he asked me to please keep him apprised of what was going on. I promised him I would and hung up.

After that call, Mom went back to calling out to Dank and Biney. Then she started praying the Lord's Prayer. The first time, she said it perfectly. Each subsequent time she struggled with the words and asked me to help her. Then she shocked me by saying she wanted to go home to Mississippi to see Nettie and her mom. She had not mentioned them once during the last two months, other than when she thought I was Nettie. What did this represent? Did it represent anything at all, or was I just reading too much into it?

Mom had no desire to sit up or get out of bed all day long. She also had no desire for food. When Daniel came home, she heard the door and asked, "Is that Daniel?" When I said it was, she told him to come where she could see him, which he did. She smiled, raised her arms, and said, "I'm ready to get up." It was as if a light had come on.

He put on his gloves and told her to grab him. She surprised us both by saying, "No get up." As soon as he took off the gloves, she wanted to get up again. He then asked if she wanted shrimp, and she said yes. I just had to laugh. It was magical to witness the relationship they had. Beautiful! She had refused food all day, and now she wanted shrimp? While Daniel went to prepare it it, she tried to pray again and asked for my help. I wrote the words to the Lord's Prayer on a piece of paper, using a heavy black marker, and taped it on her wall within easy view for her. My hope was that she would look at it whenever she wanted to pray and couldn't remember the words. Instead, she ripped it down again and again until I stopped taping it up. I stayed with her until Nicholas arrived and then returned home to George.

Wednesday was a good day for Mom. She woke up in a pleasant mood and was cooperative with Meisha. She wanted to get up, so Meisha dressed her, put her in her wheelchair, and moved her to the living room, where she watched television. Meisha sent me a photo of Mom sitting and snacking while watching television, and I spontaneously smiled. Mom remained downstairs until the hospice aide came. She mentioned that her feet and legs hurt, so she was given medication for pain and helped back into bed.

Mom refused care as usual and called for Dank until she went to sleep. She remained calm until Meisha left, and Daniel stated that Mom remained in bed for the remainder of the evening. I'm sure the act of getting up and being moved to the living room had taken a toll on her. Daniel said Mom continued to speak of Dank and Biney throughout the evening, but he had not wanted to medicate her because she was calm and not showing any signs of distress. She awakened at 2:00 a.m. Thursday morning somewhat agitated, so she was given medication at that time. Both she and Daniel slept through the night after that.

On Thursday, I received several calls from Meisha regarding Mom's behavior. Mom was being verbally and physically abusive, calling her names and kicking and hitting her. She was also throwing anything within her reach at Meisha. I asked Meisha if she could identify anything that had happened before Mom's tirade that may have precipitated the behavior, but she couldn't. I told her to try to give her the antianxiety medication and let me know whether that helped. Then came the call that Mom had fallen, and Meisha couldn't get her up. I called Don to come help her.

Lesson: When someone with dementia acts out, you may be able to identify something that happened just before the negative behavior. Tracking this in a journal could prove useful in helping you determine what not to do to avoid a particular behavior.

While I was on the phone with Don, Meisha called back to inform me she had been able to get Mom off the floor and had given her the antianxiety medication. Don was at the bowling alley when I called him, so I asked if he could please stop by Mom's on his way home to make sure all was well. He told me he would. An hour later, Meisha called back to advise me that Mom had settled down. Thank God, I thought. I always held my breath when Meisha was having a rough time with Mom. When would she reach her breaking point? She'd assured me that she would not quit because she needed the money, but I wondered sometimes how much one person could take.

Meisha and Mom had both survived what I felt had been their worst day together. One more day down and God only knows how many more to go. "One day at a time, sweet Jesus. That's all I'm asking of you."

Friday was my scheduled day to spend the afternoon with Mom. Because Meisha had taken Tuesday off for personal reasons, she asked if she could work a full day on Friday. I said yes, fully understanding the importance of her having a steady income stream. I went out as planned because I was going to spend the night. I would have Meisha tend to Mom's personal needs while I continued to clean and do other things that needed to be done.

Taking a chance that Mom might have an appetite and eat something for me, I decided to stop at KFC to pick up some baked wings, mashed potatoes, and coleslaw. When I arrived at about 1:00 p.m., Mom was quiet. Reviewing the care journal, we saw she had received antianxiety medication at 3:00 a.m. Lately, the effects seemed to be lasting longer. I made a note to ask Jenna if that was common, as I expected it to become less effective over time instead of more so.

I went to Mom's room, asked if she was hungry and was shocked when she said she was. I had been smart enough this time to have the food with me, knowing that if she said yes and I went to get it, she would change her mind by the time I returned. I took the meat off the bones of the wings and held up the saucer that held her meal. She was interested in feeding herself, which was good.

Because she was having trouble using the fork, she quickly resorted to using her fingers. Even though she loved chicken, she was finished after only a couple of bites. After barely tasting the coleslaw, she wanted nothing to do with it and wouldn't even try the mashed potatoes. She had eaten the equivalent of a few forkfuls of food and clamped her mouth shut when I tried to coax her into eating more.

After she finished eating, she asked to go to bed, so Meisha and I helped her to lie down. She slept for about an hour before starting her ritual of calling deceased relatives. When I went to comfort her, she looked at me and said, "Dank's dead, isn't he?" When I told her he was, she wanted to know how he'd died. I told her I didn't know, and she became quiet as a tear rolled slowly down her cheek. Shortly thereafter, she drifted off to sleep.

Jenna arrived and Mom woke up as she was being examined. She was compliant, not yelling at Jenna or telling her to stop. When Jenna went downstairs, Mom began calling out for Nettie. After a couple of minutes, I went to her room. She looked up and asked, "Net. What took you so long?" I explained I was speaking with her nurse and asked if she needed anything. When she said she didn't know, I let her know that

I needed to go back to speak with the nurse and would be back. As I left the room, she told me to hurry back.

While going over questions and concerns with Jenna, Mom began to incessantly call Dank and Biney again. Although we had told Jenna that Mom had been doing this, this was the first time she was able to witness the extent of what we had told her. She became disturbed and said, "Would you be opposed to my giving her an Ativan?" I told her not at all and said that it was difficult to determine whether we were dealing with end-of-life issues or dementia issues. Jenna reminded me that it didn't matter. She said, "The Ativan will calm her regardless of whether it's end-of-life or dementia."

I shared Daniel's concern that Ativan had a doping effect and his hesitancy to use it. He did not want Mom to become "comatose." Jenna stated that Ativan does stay in the system for about twenty hours and that when used regularly, it would build up and result in a very lethargic patient. She stated that hospitals use a much larger dose than we were using and that they administer it intravenously. As such, persons Daniel sees in the hospital setting do appear more "comatose."

Jenna reminded me that our goal was to keep Mom comfortable, and asked how Mom could be comfortable if she was constantly calling for those who have passed on before her. Even though Mom didn't sound distressed when calling out to her relatives, I agreed that she was probably anxious. Mom was given the Ativan and it took more than an hour for the medication to take effect.

Jenna and I then had a conversation about visioning. I told her I hadn't realized visioning could go on for so long: Mom had been visioning for over a week. Jenna stated it could go on for weeks before death. When I asked if Mom was heading in that direction, she looked at me compassionately. When I told her to speak with me candidly, she stated that she felt that was the case. Mom's intake of food and fluids was still minimal, as well as her output. Her vitals were good, but there was no improvement in her condition.

177

Before Jenna left, we again reviewed medications. This had become the norm, and I realized that she felt we were underutilizing the medications. I assured her that I would have the same conversation with Daniel and that we would hopefully all get on the same page.

Later that afternoon, Don saw my car in the driveway and decided to stop by. I noticed that he would be in the room with Mom while I was there but would follow me downstairs when I'd leave the room. I wondered if he was uncomfortable being alone with Mom. I didn't get it at first, but later I did. I think I was comfortable with the idea of death because of my years of working in the hospice field. Don had never witnessed death. Yes, he had experienced losses caused by death, but this was the first time he was witnessing the process. The idea of Mom's dying process was challenging for him.

As her oldest child, Don had known Mom longer than any of us. He'd shared experiences that the rest of us had only heard about, and this would magnify his anticipatory grief. Of course he would not want to be present—and alone—at the moment of Mom's passing. Don, Daniel, Nicholas, and I all had special connections with Mom. I was her only daughter; Daniel was her primary caregiver; Nicholas was her youngest child; and Don was her eldest.

> **Lesson:** There is no right or wrong way to feel about whether to be present when someone dies.

While Don and I were in Mom's room, I mentioned how she had found and devoured the two candy bars Lena had brought her. Mom was listening and asked if she could have candy. When Don asked if he should go buy some candy for her, I told him that he should speak with Daniel first. When he did, Daniel said no. I responded that if it were up to me, she could eat whatever the hell she wanted. Don felt the same way. Daniel said that Mom had only a few teeth left and that all that candy was not good for her.

Initially, I was annoyed but then reflected on some things. As I thought back, I had a lightbulb moment. Everyone but Daniel was behaving as if Mom were dying, because Mom *was* dying. Daniel was behaving as if Mom were living, because Mom *was* living. While most of us were busy anticipating Mom's death, Daniel was busy helping her live. Everything he did was being done to preserve her life. The rest of us were focused only on keeping her comfortable until she died.

Who was right? We all were. Who was wrong? We all were. Acceptance of someone's impending death does not mean giving up and letting go. It also doesn't, in my opinion, mean pushing someone to do things that they may not want to do, or pushing them not to do things that they do want to do. I don't believe there are any right or wrong answers. We all do the best we can, in the name of love, while trying to honor our loved one in the process. People express their love differently.

Lesson: As long as expressions of love are not causing physical or emotional harm, it's all good.

Over the weekend, I called Daniel multiple times to see how Mom was doing. I left messages advising him he didn't need to call back unless there was a change, but I was hoping he'd call. He had always called back before, but not this time. Not hearing from him was driving me nuts. Was he okay? Was Mom okay? He'd call me if Mom wasn't okay, wouldn't he? If something happened to him, he wouldn't be able to call me. I could always call one of my brothers to have them check in and get back with me. Perhaps I should do that. Those were just a few of the many thoughts that ran through my mind. Finally, I realized that I was being irrational.

I had told him he didn't need to call if there was no change and needed to give him a little space. After all, I had been calling every day. I was smothering him. I didn't need to call him every single day. Meisha kept me posted daily during the week. I was with Mom on Fridays and part of the day on Saturdays. What more did I need?

I realized that I needed constant reassurance that my mom did not need me. I had complete confidence that Daniel was doing everything that Mom needed to have done. I had to trust that Daniel would call me if he or Mom needed anything. I trusted him fully and needed to back off.

Early Monday morning, Meisha called to let me know that Mom was truly giving her a run for her money, being combative and close to giving a repeat performance of last week's incidents. She said that Daniel was out of the house quickly that morning and said, "Good luck!" as he hurried out the door. That to me was an indication that he'd had a rough weekend. He should have called me, I thought. Let it go LaBena, I told myself.

I suggested that Meisha give Mom her antianxiety medication and call me back with an update in an hour and she agreed. Since I had been coming out twice weekly since her most recent hospitalization, I would be seeing Mom on Tuesday and did not feel the need to rush out. I could also see that George was concerned that Meisha was calling me so often. He was thinking that if she'd had so much experience dealing with individuals who had dementia, she shouldn't need to call me as frequently as she did. I shared that Meisha hadn't had my mom as a patient and was doing what I'd instructed her to do.

Lesson: One person with dementia is one person with dementia. The illness can manifest itself differently from one individual to the next, and not everyone reacts the same way to each intervention. You have to figure out what works for each individual.

Tuesday was a repeat of Monday. I reminded Meisha that I would be out around noon but gave her the okay to medicate Mom in the meantime. I prepared some clam chowder, which Mom used to enjoy, to take to her. I knew she probably wouldn't eat lunch, as she had stopped doing so long ago, but I hoped that she'd have it for dinner. This would keep Daniel from having to cook when he arrived home. On my way out, I checked with Meisha to see if there was anything needed and then stopped at the store to retrieve those items before arriving at Mom's house.

When I arrived, Mom was sitting on the edge of the bed. Of late, she seemed to enjoy doing that. She acknowledged my presence, although I don't believe she knew who I was. I said hello and introduced myself. She said hello, hugged me, and said she was tired. I convinced her to lie down, covered her with blankets, and within minutes, she was asleep. I then ate lunch and resorted to my stress reliever: cleaning.

When Mom awakened, she called out. When I entered the room, she thought I was Nettie. I allowed her to continue to think that, and she let me know that she was very sick and very tired. She would call out to Dank intermittently, then go back to speaking to me about how she was feeling. She told me that her legs really hurt, so I gave her a pain pill and asked if I could massage her legs. She said I could and commented that they felt better as I was doing so. I continued massaging them for a few minutes when she said, "That's fine."

She then began pulling at her clothing and the blankets. When I asked if she was too hot, she said yes, but then she would say she was cold. I took off the sweatshirt she was wearing, replaced it with a T-shirt, pulled the covers up to her chin, and asked if that was better. She nodded, relaxed, and began to speak.

She looked at me and asked, "Do you know when I'm going to die?" I told her that I did not and then asked if she was ready to die. She shook her head no. She told me again that she was very sick and very tired. That broke my heart because I didn't know what to do to make her feel better. I just stroked her head and held her hand.

Jenna came by and checked Mom's vitals. Although they were all within normal range, Mom's feet were cold, and her legs were blotchy. We weren't sure whether the discolored legs were part of the dying process or because she'd been kicking at things while trying to get out of bed.

While we were discussing her decline, Mom began calling Dank again. Jenna indicated that this would be a good time to give her Ativan and reiterated the purpose of the medication. We also discussed allowing Meisha to administer medications from the Comfort Care kit. I stated that I never wanted her to administer morphine but was not opposed to her administering the other medications, so long as she spoke with me first. I said I would discuss this with Daniel to secure his agreement.

By the time Daniel came home, Mom was calm and wanted to sit up. But as he was getting her up, she changed her mind. As he was laying her back down, she changed her mind yet again, so we decided to get her up and see if she would eat something. I heated the chowder I had brought, adding a couple of crackers and a few pieces of melon to her plate. She first grabbed and ate a piece of melon. When I gave her the first spoonful of chowder, she said, "That ain't nothin'!" Ouch!

Daniel asked if I had salted the chowder; I had not because I thought the bacon I'd used provided plenty of salt. He went to retrieve the saltshaker while Mom continued to eat the chowder . . . even though it wasn't "nothin'." She ended up eating about half a cup of chowder, two small bites of melon, and one cracker. Although that wasn't much, it was more than I'd seen her eat in a long time. I knew that the need for food and water diminished as death neared; I just didn't like it. It was a reminder that death wasn't far away. I knew that soon she would not eat or drink. I just wasn't ready.

Daniel returned with the salt, which we didn't need, and I spoke with him regarding Meisha being permitted to administer medications from the Comfort Care kit. He said, "If she needs the meds, she needs the meds." Progress!

When Mom finished eating, I had Daniel get her back into bed. I could see how tired she was and continued to sit with her while Daniel went to exercise. I was glad I was there to give him a break. He would typically come home, fix her dinner, and ensure she ate something, not taking time for himself until she was sound asleep.

After she finished eating, I stayed for about two hours and noticed a change. Mom was now speaking about both parents, Nettie, and her sister Addie, who had died as an infant. She said she wanted to go home. When I asked where home was, she said, "Anding, Mississippi." Her cousin Nina had previously shared with me that when she was younger, Mom had spent quite a bit of time in Anding doing whatever she wanted to do. It was obvious that Mom had fond memories of Anding. No wonder she would want to return there.

Once she was settled and Daniel had done everything he wanted and needed to do, I went home. It was much easier leaving her knowing she was resting well.

About 9:00 a.m. the following day, I received a call from Meisha stating that Mom was agitated and uncooperative. I asked her to put the phone to Mom's ear and asked what was wrong. "I'm very sick and I don't feel well," Mom said. When I asked what was wrong, she said, "My stomach hurts real bad." I told her to hold on and that I would have Meisha give her something to make her feel better.

I called hospice, relaying what my mom had told me and requesting a recommendation for medication to relieve her stomach pain. Jenna told us to try the anti-nausea medication first, and if that didn't help, try giving her Mylanta. She volunteered to come to the house if we needed her to. I let her know I would call if her suggested remedies weren't effective. Then I called Meisha, advising her to give Mom the anti-nausea medication. I also called Nicholas to have him pick up Mylanta to take to the house. Even if the anti-nausea medication was helpful this time, I thought it would be a good idea to have Mylanta on hand for the next time. I then had Meisha give the Ativan to Mom to relax her.

Fortunately, the anti-nausea medication, coupled with the Ativan, seemed to help. Mom's stomach pain resolved and she was able to rest for the remainder of the afternoon. I was pleased with the outcome, as was Meisha.

Unfortunately, with dementia, success can be short-lived. Meisha called bright and early Thursday morning to tell me that Mom had slid out of her wheelchair and, because Mom was combative, she was unable to get her up and into the bed. Meisha had tried to give her Ativan, but Mom wouldn't take it. I told her to make sure Mom was sitting comfortably on the floor, stay with her, and I would have Don come over to assist.

I called Don, who immediately went over. He was able to get Mom into bed and eventually convinced her to take her medications. I was grateful that my siblings continued to help when needed. Working as a cohesive unit makes difficult situations so much more manageable, especially when there is no drama involved. George felt the lack of drama was because I was dealing with men instead of women. Chauvinist!

That day, I was anxious to see Mom. She'd been having a rougher time than was her norm, and I just needed to put my eyes on her. I had made a great beef roast that was so tender it was falling apart, and I felt that she would possibly eat some of it. Because she was eating less, I wanted her to fully enjoy whatever she did eat.

When I relieved Meisha, I immediately went to Mom's room to say hello. She looked up at me and said, "Lady, would you please leave me alone?" I said, "Mom, it's me, LaBena." She turned towards me, stared, and said, "LaBena?" When I said yes, she reached her arms out to me. I bent down to kiss her; she kissed me and wrapped her arms around my neck. I can't begin to tell you how that felt. I had not experienced such a showing of affection from her in a very long time. She had been recognizing me less, my heart breaking each time she looked at me blankly. I knew what was coming and tried to mentally prepare myself.

Lesson: It's a good idea to introduce yourself whenever you are visiting someone with dementia. If you are going to be providing care, you should also advise them of what you plan to do. Put yourself in their shoes. Would you like a stranger entering your private space and putting their hands on you?

As time went on, Mom became increasingly restless. She would go from trying to remove her clothing to trying to get out of bed to constantly calling out for Dank, Lucky, her mom, and her dad. No matter what I said, I was unable to comfort her. Remembering what Jenna had said and knowing that the Ativan she had been given earlier was proving ineffective, I decided to give her some morphine. This was a big move for me. I knew Mom's behavior could well be a sign of pain that she was unable to communicate, and Jenna had been encouraging me to begin using the morphine in the Comfort Care kit.

After administering the morphine, I was expecting to see a dramatic change in Mom but such was not the case. Her immediate response was, "Don't give me any more of that shit!" After an hour, Mom went to sleep for about fifteen minutes. When she woke up, she was still pulling at her clothes and trying to get out of bed. However, she was no longer crying out. I was able to engage with her and speak with her about why she was taking her clothes off and where she was going. We had a very pleasant conversation. I guess the morphine had an impact on her after all.

Lesson: Remembering the regression that occurs with persons who have dementia, I was reminded of how small children love to take off their clothes and run around. After all, she was only three!

I realized that Mom was thinking I was her sister, Nettie. When I began speaking to Mom as if I were Nettie, we were both comforted. She loved her big sister and felt safe with her. I listened to her speak about a variety of things from her youth. She even laughed out loud at one point, which was an extremely rare occurrence these days. This was a very pleasant experience.

That moment was short-lived because she became agitated again, calling out for Dank nonstop. I couldn't calm her. She began trying to climb out of bed even though I was sitting right next to her and speaking with her. Then she began hallucinating, seeing animals and people that were upsetting her. "There's a snake on the floor. What's that on the wall? Where did that cat go?" She also began to again complain about pain in her legs and feet. The medication seemed to be ineffective, so I needed to try something different.

As I had done before, I asked if I could massage her legs, which she agreed to and seemed to find comforting. Suddenly she asked me to stop, stating that I was hurting her. I then gave her both her pain and antianxiety medications, which the nurse had instructed me to do. She took the pills without hesitation as I continued speaking to her in what I hoped was a soothing manner. After a while, I gently stroked her head, thinking it would help calm her. Instead, she said, "Will you please stop rubbing my head?" I stopped immediately, and about five minutes later, Mom drifted off to sleep.

When Daniel came home, he could tell that Mom had been medicated, and I don't think he was happy about it. I explained how she had behaved during the day and told him that was why she had received so many of her medications. He didn't respond. I had learned previously that Mom was a different person in Daniel's presence; I'd not seen her become agitated or angry with him. Instead, she tended to become submissive and childlike. Daniel was bald and had dark brown skin. Her dad had been bald and had dark brown skin. Was she thinking Daniel was her dad? Who knows? What I do know is that there was a special bond between the two of them, and it was an absolute pleasure to witness their interactions.

I thought back fondly to a conversation Mom and I had had over one of our lunches. She was speaking about her father, how much he loved her, and how much he let her get away with. She had said that when she did something wrong, "He only whupped me for show so Net wouldn't get jealous." Nina had confirmed Mom's stories saying that Grandpa let Mom get away with everything.

I stayed over that night, and Mom slept eighteen hours without waking up. It was as if all the medications were kicking in at one time. Then I recalled Jenna telling me that the medications build up in the system with regular use. Because she was sleeping so soundly, Daniel entrusted me with her care while he exercised. When Mom awakened, the first word out of her mouth was "Candy." Even though I knew Daniel probably wouldn't approve, I gave her a piece of a Baby Ruth bar I had seen. As it turned out, Daniel had a stash of Baby Ruth bars put away for her. He wasn't so tough after all, I thought. It took quite a while for her to eat her candy, but she was very satisfied afterward.

Lesson: The taste buds of a person with dementia, as well as the elderly in general, can change over time. Salt and sweet seem to be what they are most able to taste, which may have accounted for Mom's increased desire for sweets.

Because she appeared to be doing so well, I decided it was a good time to try to give Mom a bed bath. Both her hospice caregiver and Meisha had been unable to do so earlier in the week, so I wanted to see if I could. I did! Mom was cooperative as I bathed her. It was such a humbling experience for me, and tears welled up in my eyes. This woman had been so strong. She was aware of what I was doing, and I knew, if she were in her right mind, she'd hate that I was doing this. She was defeated, and I noticed tears in her eyes as well. I am sure she felt better once the bath was completed; however, she seemed sad.

Daniel finished exercising and returned to Mom's room with a shampoo cap. I had never seen or heard of a shampoo cap before. It resembled a regular shower cap but had a special lining that was filled with no-rinse shampoo. The cap is heated in the microwave and then placed on the head; the shampoo is massaged into the scalp and the cap is removed. The result is clean hair.

Mom's reaction was similar to that of a puppy when you rub its tummy or scratch it behind the ears. She turned her head toward whatever area I was massaging, having an ever so slight smile on her face. You could tell she was enjoying the experience, although she didn't utter a word.

After the bath and shampoo, Mom fell asleep again and I decided to take the opportunity to speak with Daniel about Mom's finances. Although Daniel was her financial power of attorney and attorney-in-fact, I was her financial manager. I was the one who paid all the bills and monitored spending from her account. I let Daniel know how much money was in Mom's bank account, how much came in monthly, and what her regular monthly expenses were. We had not had to go into Mom's savings as yet, but I thought that time might not be too far off.

Lesson: It's a good idea to maintain a spreadsheet listing all expenses, account numbers, due dates, etc., to ensure all bills are paid on time in the event someone becomes incapacitated.

Daniel then surprised me by saying that he was sure we would not have to go into her savings and hoped he was not jinxing things by saying that out loud. What? How was the guy we thought was in denial about Mom's condition making the statement—while not making the statement—that Mom would not be around long enough for us to have to go into her savings to pay her expenses?

As we spoke further, it was obvious that Daniel was very much aware that Mom's life expectancy was short. What I came to realize was that Daniel did not want to hear what others had to say about her condition because he was not going to let what others thought have any bearing on how he chose to care for Mom. Again, while others were waiting for Mom to die, he was busy helping her live her best life for as long as that life was. Wasn't that the hospice philosophy? He was dealing with Mom's condition in a much healthier way than I was. I so admired him!

When I was ready to leave and got to my car, I realized I had left something in Mom's room and went back into the house. I was shocked to see that she had urinated—a lot. She had not passed urine in about five days, so I was stunned and happy. Perhaps all that buildup of urine had been the reason for her discomfort, anxiety, and pain. Could she have cheated death again? Was this yet another sign that it was not yet her time?

When I left that Saturday, I was smiling. My mom could not have a better primary caregiver. I just needed to trust Daniel more. That meant that I had to stop calling every night to see how she was doing. I had to trust that he would call me with any pertinent changes in Mom's condition and that he would let me know if he needed assistance. I know I'd said all of this before, but this time I meant it. I didn't call him that night or the following day.

Early Monday morning, Meisha called me stating that Mom was picking out her funeral flowers. I told her to let me speak with Mom, and she put the phone on speaker, initially trying to coax Mom into repeating what she had told her. I told Meisha to let Mom speak as I began to talk to her.

"It's LaBena, Mom. What are you doing?" I asked.

"Picking flowers," she replied.

"Why are you picking flowers?" I asked.

"For my funeral," she said.

"Do you think you are going to die?"

189

"Everybody is going to die sometime," she responded.

I laughed. "Are you ready to die?"

"No," she replied.

"What kind of flowers are you picking?" I asked.

"Pink ones," she said.

"What kind of pink ones?"

"I don't know," she responded.

"You've always liked roses and carnations," I said.

"Pink carnations," she said.

"That's nice," I said. "Enjoy picking your flowers. I'll speak to you later. I love you."

Silence. Before hanging up, I thanked Meisha for calling and asked her to let me know if she noticed any other unusual behaviors. I thought back to Mom's funeral preparations. She had picked out a beautiful pink casket with a blue floral arrangement stitched into the inside lining. Although I had never seen Mom wear pink, it was obviously one of her favorite colors. Heck, although my favorite color was yellow, I didn't own one piece of yellow clothing.

While making a mental note that Mom wanted pink carnations at her funeral, I also recalled a conversation we had after attending the funeral of one of her friends. "I want my flowers while I am alive," she had said. I decided to bring Mom pink carnations when I next visited her.

I planned on visiting on Tuesday and Friday, but Meisha needed Wednesday afternoon off. As such, I would be visiting on Wednesday and Friday. I spoke with Jenna on Tuesday after her visit, and she again reviewed medications and the need to keep Mom comfortable. I also shared that Mom had urinated on Saturday, but that output had been minimal since then. She stated that she would come back on Friday to reassess her and that we would speak further at that time.

On Wednesday morning, Meisha called saying Mom was agitated again. I instructed her to give Mom an Ativan and let me know in about an hour whether it was effective. She called an hour later to say that Mom was even more agitated, trying to get out of bed and taking her clothes off. Jenna had previously instructed us to give her another dose if that happened, which I had Meisha do. Before hanging up, I reminded her that I would be there between 11:30 a.m. and noon.

I sautéed some shrimp and made a small sweet potato soufflé, just in case Mom desired something to eat. On my way out, I stopped by the Honey Baked Ham store to pick up a sandwich and some chips for me to eat for lunch. I then stopped and purchased pink carnations for her.

When I reached Mom's house, she was still showing some signs of agitation, calling out and trying to get out of bed. However, she seemed to recognize me and smiled when she saw me. I leaned in to kiss her, and she kissed me back. This was a rarity. I was pretending that she knew I was her daughter, although I was pretty sure she thought I was her sister. When I showed her the flowers, she said, "They pretty."

I asked Mom if she was hungry, and to my surprise, she said yes. I went and warmed her food and returned to the room. She ate two shrimp (and no sweet potato soufflé) before announcing she was done. I knew not to ask her to try to eat more, although I wanted her to.

I sat and tried to speak with Mom, but she did not respond. Because I was hungry, I decided to get my lunch and sit with her while I ate. As I was eating, I noticed Mom staring at my bag of chips. Suddenly she said, "Give me one of those chips." Shocked, I handed her a chip. She ate it and asked for another . . . and then another. After three chips, she announced she was finished. Although it was only three chips, it made me smile. Why did seeing her eat make me so happy? Perhaps it's because many of us view the sharing of food as an expression of love.

Lesson: In many cultures, food is a major focus of family celebrations and is how we show love. Perhaps that is why we try to encourage people to continue to eat even when their bodies are telling them they are dying and no longer need food.

When I finished eating, Mom looked at me and asked, "When do we need to be at the train station?" Here we go with the hospice speak, I thought.

Lesson: Oftentimes, persons nearing the end of life will speak of packing bags and taking trips. It had always amazed me when I would read or hear about the occurrences of this phenomenon.

Mom did not want us to miss the train. Suddenly, she began saying "teddy bear" repeatedly. I asked if she wanted a teddy bear, and she said she didn't. I knew she was trying to communicate something, but I couldn't figure out what it was. Perhaps she'd had a favorite teddy bear as a child and wanted to be sure to take it on her trip. When I told Lynn and Ann about Mom's mentioning of the teddy bear, they made sure I had one to give her when I visited again.

After a short time, Mom fell asleep peacefully and seemed to be at rest when Daniel came home from work. He tried to encourage me to leave, but I told him I was fine staying with Mom until he completed his workout. He finally relented. While he was working out, Nicholas stopped by. Mom had since awakened but was withdrawn. She didn't respond to much of anything and appeared to be sad.

Nicholas tried to convince me to leave, stating he would stay with Mom until Daniel completed his workout. Initially, I didn't want to go, but I had another lightbulb moment. Others wanted to spend quality time with Mom just as I did. I realized that my staying would have deprived Nicholas of his time with her. To do so would make me selfish. I left in order to give Nicholas private time with her, knowing I would have more time with her on Friday.

Early Friday morning, I received a call from Jenna advising me she was ill and would not be able to check in on Mom. She took a verbal update from me, offered suggestions for any concerns I had, and offered to have another nurse complete a home visit. I declined that offer. We also decided to release the hospice aide assigned to Mom from her duties because Mom never allowed her to provide any care. After Jenna stated she would check in on Mom early in the following week, I hung up. Since Jenna wouldn't be coming by, I decided to go to Ravenna later in the day.

Mom did not recognize me initially, saying, "Lady would you please leave me alone and get out of my house?" I know I should have introduced myself, but instead slowly leaned in closer without saying a word. She looked at me and started laughing. "LaBena, I didn't know who you were," she said. Although she had given Meisha a rough time earlier in the day, she was pleasant toward me. She said she was hungry but ate and drank nothing when I brought her lunch to her.

I let Meisha leave early, per her request, and sat with Mom. Suddenly, she thought I was Nettie again. "Where are Mommy and Daddy?" she asked. "Are they coming home soon?" I let her know that she would see them soon, which I really believed. Then she asked for Dank and Lucky. After a while, she became sleepy and I recalled that earlier, Meisha had given her medication for pain and anxiety. Obviously, the medication was beginning to kick in.

Abruptly, Mom became alert and asked, "Who are those two ladies?" When I asked what ladies, she said, "The ones standing right beside you. I don't know who they are, and I don't think they're nice." She then yelled, "Get out!" while looking in my direction but not at me. I asked if she wanted me to leave and she said, "No. I just want that cat by your feet to leave." She was hallucinating again! Once she calmed down and fell asleep, I went downstairs and thought back to the two ladies she had just seen. I wondered if they had been her mom and sister, but she had not recognized them. Dementia is a strange beast, and it can't be turned on and off. Could it be that Mom could only visualize her mom and sister the way they had looked when she was a small child as opposed to the way they had looked when they died?

Lesson: As the person with dementia regresses, so do their memories. It is not uncommon for them to remember people the way they used to look as opposed to their current appearance. They may think their daughter is their wife, or their son is their husband. Facilities specializing in dementia care will oftentimes cover, or not have, mirrors because residents don't recognize themselves and become alarmed by the stranger looking back at them.

Mom settled down and then began repeating, "Holy, Holy, Holy." It took me a while, but I remembered that was a song that was sung at her church. I had her Echo Dot play it in an attempt to comfort her. After a minute, Mom said, "Nettie B., You singing?" I replied, "Yes, Lottie Mae. I'm singing." She smiled as she listened to the song, finally drifting off to sleep. She would awaken for a brief period of time every couple of hours thereafter, but then fall asleep again. This was becoming a pattern, with Mom sleeping more than she would be awake.

For I know the thoughts that I think toward you, saith the Lord, thoughts of peace, and not of evil, to give you an expected end.
Jeremiah 29:11

Chapter 21
A Closer Walk

Nineteen Days Post-Ninety!

We began to see yet another change in Mom's urinary habits, with her urinating only once per week for the past couple of weeks. She was dehydrated, and we had been told that Mom was in kidney failure. That made sense. Why else would someone urinate only once per week? That pattern broke on Saturday when I went into Mom's room and was shocked to be greeted by the smell of urine. When I checked the bed, Mom was covered from head to toe with urine. It was as if a dam had burst and the floodwaters came rushing through. Was this a good or a bad thing? Did this mean she was not in kidney failure? Again, Mom had surprised us.

Lesson: Expect the unexpected.

After Daniel and I gave Mom a bed bath and changed her bed, she suddenly asked, "Who preached at Simon's funeral?" I had no idea who Simon was and couldn't respond to her question. She asked again and became upset with me when I didn't know the answer.

Once Mom had calmed down, something told me to ask her to tell me the names of her children. She said, "Don, Lewis, John, LaBena, Daniel, Simon, and Nicholas." I waited a bit and again asked her to name her children. She repeated the names just as she had before. This was interesting because, to my knowledge, I did not have a brother named Simon. Andrew, who had died at the age of two, had been born between the births of Daniel and Nicholas; she hadn't mentioned his name.

Andrew, my dad, and John III were the only deceased relatives I had not heard Mom call out for yet. She may have done so when others were around, but not in my presence. Now she was asking questions about Simon and telling me that Simon was her son. That was a puzzle I wanted to solve, but I doubted that I would be able to do so. For now, Simon would remain an unsolved mystery.

Another mystery was the fact that she had recently stopped calling for Dank and Biney, whose names she had been calling relentlessly. Now she was only asking for her mom, her dad, and her sister Nettie. Although her sister Addie had died as an infant, she never called for her. I wondered if the fact that Addie and Andrew had both been infants when they died was the reason she never called for them. I would never know the answer to that question.

Whenever Mom asked for her parents, I would tell her that she'd see them soon. She was now consistently referring to me as Nettie B., which I treasured. The night before, she had asked if she could sleep in my bed. I told her my room was a mess and offered to stay with her until she fell asleep, which was an offer she gratefully accepted. Somehow, being thought of as her sister made the pain of her no longer knowing me as her daughter a little easier to handle.

While preparing her breakfast that Saturday morning, I heard Mom crying out, "Nettie B." When I reached her room and asked what she needed, she said, "What took you so long?" I told her I was fixing her breakfast; she replied that she wasn't hungry. Thinking I was her sister was a source of comfort to Mom and to me.

Mom appeared to be wide awake for a change, although not at all talkative. Remembering how much she used to enjoy westerns, I scanned her television with hopes of finding *Bonanza* or some other western I knew she once enjoyed watching. She smiled when I happened upon *Walker, Texas Ranger*, and actually said the words. I sat silently watching the show with her.

She was surprisingly attentive to the show and occasionally offered a one- or two-word comment. When it was time for me to leave, Daniel went into the room to sit and watch the show with her. It did my soul good to see her so relaxed. When I let her know I was leaving, she asked for greens and cornbread again. Knowing she wouldn't eat it if I prepared it that day, I told her I would bring some to her the next time I came. When I brought some soup up for her to eat, she said she wasn't hungry. I told her I loved her and waited for the response I so craved, but it wasn't to be.

When I returned on Tuesday, collard greens and cornbread in hand as promised, Mom surprised me by attempting to eat them. I say attempted because she would put some in her mouth, chew and chew, and never swallow. I finally asked her if she needed to spit the food out, to which she nodded her head yes. I held a tissue to her mouth as she spat a wad of spent greens into it.

Lesson: Persons with dementia can reach a point where they forget how to chew and swallow and may require a little coaching and guidance in order to do so.

I wondered if Mom had not swallowed her food because she had forgotten how. I was not to know the answer to that question.

Thirty Days Post-Ninety!

On the morning of Wednesday, May 2, I received a call from Meisha advising me that something seemed wrong with Mom's breathing. When I asked what she meant, she said, "She's just not breathing right." She had already called Jenna, who was on her way, but wanted me to know what was going on. I asked her to have Jenna call me once she arrived and assessed Mom.

After about twenty minutes, I received a call from Jenna telling me that I'd better come. I let George know what was going on, packed a bag, and once again headed to Ravenna. I was surprised I was able to hold it together as I drove, but my mind kept going back to how many times Mom had been at death's door and rallied back. Perhaps this would be another one of those times, I thought. But then I wondered how many times she could possibly continue to do so.

While in the car, I called and left messages for each of my brothers, advising them of what had occurred. I arrived at Mom's and was met by Meisha, who was visibly shaken. Mom had aspirated on some water and had been having trouble breathing since that time. When I reached her room, Mom instantly perked up. She even smiled at me, although she didn't say anything. Jenna motioned for me to follow her downstairs.

When we reached the dining room, Jenna let me know the time was very close and that she was putting Mom on watch, which meant a nurse would be coming by every day to check on her. When she reached the point that they felt death was imminent, she would be placed into the Even More program, and someone from Crossroads would be present continuously until she died. I told her I didn't know how Daniel would feel about that but that we would cross that bridge when we came to it.

Don came over shortly after I'd arrived, with Daniel and Nicholas both coming after they got off work. Mom was resting comfortably when they arrived. Although she spoke very little, she was responsive to us. When she drifted off to sleep, we all convened in the living room to discuss what we felt might be happening soon. I think we were all completely ready to accept what was happening and were feeling bad for what we saw as the length of Mom's suffering. We agreed that she seemed tired and ready to go.

I stayed overnight and before going to bed, I whispered to Mom, "It's okay to go if you are ready. We will be okay, and I promise we will look out for each other." Daniel and I slept little that night. It was as if he and I were on a clock that told us when to get up and check on Mom.

In earlier years, I recalled Mom speaking about hoping she would die in her sleep. That thought kept resonating with me throughout the night, which is why I kept getting up to check her breathing. I'm sure Daniel was doing the same.

Lesson: Through my hospice experiences, I learned that oftentimes someone nearing death needs permission from their loved ones to die. They may also hold on due to some type of unfinished business. Perhaps they are waiting to see someone, or have a need to hear something from someone, before they are ready to pass on.

Thirty-One Days Post-Ninety!

On Thursday, Mom seemed to have rallied once again, and I wondered why she was holding on. She had seen or spoken to everyone she'd had a desire to see or speak to, and I had assured her that we would continue to look out for each other. Whatever the reason, it was obvious she was not ready to go.

Jenna arrived and conducted an assessment. She looked at me and said, "All of your Mom's vitals are normal. I don't know what's happening, but we are going to take her off watch." I told her that Mom, for some reason, was just not ready to go. Since she was doing so well, I decided to leave her in Meisha's care and go home.

Because I had already stayed over on Wednesday, I hadn't planned to go to Ravenna on Friday. However, I awakened with an overwhelming need to see Mom. As if on cue, Meisha called stating that Mom was in pain and asking what she should do. I asked her to look in the journal and let me know when Mom had last received pain medication. She told me that Daniel had given Mom antianxiety medication before going to work, but no pain medication had been administered. Hearing this, I instructed her to administer the pain medication and told her that I would be making an unplanned trip to Ravenna within a couple of hours.

George decided to ride with me this time since I wasn't planning to stay overnight. I was hesitant at first, thinking I'd be staying over if I needed to. I then decided I could still stay over; he'd just need to either stay with me or come pick me up on Saturday or whenever.

When we arrived and went to Mom's room, her breathing was labored. Despite that, she refused her oxygen. When I tried to convince her that she would feel better with the oxygen, she said nastily, "I told you I don't want that!" I told her that I understood she didn't feel well but that was not an excuse to be so mean.

George tried to make conversation with Mom, but she wasn't interested. Because of her behavior, I decided to stay until Daniel got home from work and advised Meisha that she could leave. She looked relieved. I deduced that Meisha may have been scared to be present if and when Mom died. Just because someone has cared for the elderly for years does not mean that they have been present for their deaths. At that moment, I felt I had a better understanding of why she had been calling me so frequently. I had been her reassurance that she wouldn't be alone if something happened to Mom.

Mom seemed tired by the time Daniel arrived home, so George and I made sure they didn't need anything and decided to go home. I kissed her, told her I loved her and said that I would see her soon. I never would have guessed that would be the last time I'd see my mother alive.

Thirty-Three Days Post-Ninety!

The call came at 12:45 a.m. on May 5. I knew before I answered that it would be Daniel telling me that Mom was dead, and I was right. "She's gone," he said. She's gone! For more than ten years I'd witnessed Alzheimer's and vascular dementia whittle away at Mom's mind, body, and spirit. For more than ten years I'd struggled with the emotional roller coaster that Mom, my siblings, and I had been riding. For more than ten years I'd dreaded this very moment and now everything had been summed up in two words: she's gone. She's gone. That's it? No more trips to the hospital. No more calls from Meisha. No more calls from Mom. No more being a caregiver . . . because she's gone.

Wasn't it just like Mom, the beer lover, to die on Cinco de Mayo? Although I tried not to, I began to sob uncontrollably. I thought I was prepared, but how could a daughter ever truly be prepared to say goodbye to her mother? She's gone.

George and I got out of bed, dressed, and drove in silence to Mom's home. When we arrived, Don, Nicholas, and Daniel were sitting in the living room. I felt that John and Lewis should have been there; perhaps they were. As each of my brothers rose to hug me, I collapsed into their arms. A hospice aide was in Mom's room preparing to bathe her once the nurse pronounced her time of death. She's really gone.

I went up to say goodbye to Mom. Although extremely sad, I was also comforted by the fact that she was finally at peace. She had truly fought the good fight over these past few months. Looking at her, I felt an overwhelming need to assist with her bathing. I'm not sure why I felt I wanted, or would be able, to do this. How could I even consider this? I didn't know why or how, but I knew it was something I needed to do.

As the aide began to bathe Mom's lower extremities, I cleansed her upper area. Feeling so extremely close to Mom, it was like a spiritual experience. Then I messed up. I couldn't understand why suds were forming in my mom's hair until I realized I had grabbed the regular instead of the no-rinse shampoo.

I began to laugh before breaking down into hysterical sobs. I could almost hear my mom fussing at me for messing up her hair. I could also imagine her telling me to go away and let the professional do her job. I decided (to the pleasure of the aide and Mom, I'm sure) to leave the remaining task of bathing Mom to the aide. I returned downstairs and did not recount my mishap to my brothers or to George.

The nurse contacted the funeral home to come for Mom's body, and we sat quietly while awaiting their arrival. Once they arrived, they advised us that someone would be in touch with us later in the day to discuss details. When they left, Nicholas, Don, and I made sure Daniel was okay. We told him we'd contact our own immediate families. I also volunteered to contact Lewis' kids, and said I'd reach out to our cousin Ronnie to ask her to contact the extended family on the Berry side and Nina to reach out to the Polk side. Then Don, Nicholas, and George and

I went on our way. I didn't like leaving Daniel alone but knew this was something he would get used to, perhaps much sooner than he'd like.

When George and I arrived home at about 4:00 a.m., I had no desire to go to bed. George convinced me that I needed to try to go to sleep, knowing how stressful the coming day(s) would be and that I badly needed the rest. I suggested that I would just stay downstairs and rest on the couch, but he insisted that I go up to the bedroom, change clothes, and go to bed, which I eventually conceded to do.

I lay in bed until about 8:00 a.m., then got up, showered, and dressed. At about nine thirty, I decided it would be okay to begin making calls. I first called Lynn. She heard my voice and immediately knew what had happened. We both began to sob as I shared the events of the week with her. Suddenly, a cardinal appeared on the banister of my deck and stayed there, seeming to look right into the window at me. I started laughing and said, "Mom sent a cardinal to let me know she is okay."

> **Lesson:** Many people believe that cardinals are messengers from deceased loved ones, letting them know they are fine and thinking of them.

I could not recall seeing cardinals in my yard before, even though I'm sure they had always been there. I'd never noticed them before. We both waited silently for the cardinal to leave. I was so comforted by the visit. I didn't care that the idea of cardinals bringing messages from deceased loved ones was superstition. It meant the world to me, and I wouldn't have traded that moment for anything.

Lynn wanted to come over, but I told her I would be headed back to Ravenna shortly. She asked what I needed her to do, and I responded that almost everything had been done in advance. I wanted to make calls to Lewis's kids, Leigh and Anthony, because I maintained a good relationship with both of them and wanted them to hear the news from me. I also called Mom's cousin Nina and my cousin Ronnie so they could notify extended family members.

My brothers and I agreed to ask everyone to please not post anything to social media for at least twenty-four hours. We wanted to have ample opportunity to reach out to people personally instead of learning of Mom's death on Facebook. Unfortunately, someone (who was not even related) decided to use Facebook as a means to express sympathy for our loss. I had hoped we had reached all family members personally before that post appeared, but I didn't know for sure.

Since neither Daniel nor I had heard from the funeral home by the time they'd told us we should be contacted, I decided to call them. The director said that he'd been busy all morning meeting with another family, but when I told him my siblings wanted to have the service no later than Wednesday, he agreed to meet with us that day. Nicholas and Daniel were still working and had only a few days available for funeral leave. Understandably, they did not want to take time off, go back to work, and then take more time off.

My brothers did not want things to drag on, although I was stressed thinking about having to get a funeral together in such a short amount of time. Then I remembered that there was little for us to do. When I offered a half-hearted objection to moving so fast, stating that people wouldn't have time to make travel or work arrangements, I was reminded that Mom's friends were all retired and lived locally. Most of the relatives she spoke with regularly were elderly and probably not going to travel anyhow. I conceded. They were right.

Later that day, as we sat with the funeral director, he let us know that they had no problem having the funeral on the upcoming Wednesday, but he needed to make sure the church and the people Mom wanted to officiate were available. He then began asking us a series of questions about Mom when I asked, "Are you writing her obituary?" He said he was, and I said that it was already written. My brothers had reviewed it and any necessary changes had already been made. The funeral director said that he'd need it by first thing Monday morning;

when I said that I had it in the car, he looked surprised. I then reminded him that Mom had wanted everything done in advance.

I let him know that I also had the burial clothing she'd selected and that the only things we needed were to finalize things with the church and plan her repast. He advised us that since she had been a member of Immaculate Conception Church, he was sure Mom's repast could be held there. The advantage would be that the church would supply the food and that we could make a donation on Mom's behalf as a thank you. Knowing how much Mom had loved her church, we knew that she would have been pleased to have the repast there, but we weren't sure about the food that might be provided for guests.

Shortly thereafter, the funeral director received a call back from Reverend Pierce advising us that Wednesday would be fine for the funeral and asking us to hold the repast there as well. He said, "Your Mom was a beloved member, and we'd like you to hold the repast at the church." At that point, we hadn't made our final decision about the repast. The reality was that the congregation of Immaculate Conception was about ninety-nine percent Caucasian. Would they provide the type of food that would be pleasing to our predominantly African American family members and friends? We needed to ponder this decision a little longer.

Mom had already chosen her casket during her preplanning. Unfortunately, the pink casket with its pale blue satin lining she had selected was no longer being manufactured. This was upsetting to me. She wanted her pink casket, and I wanted to honor her wish. Now I couldn't because it was not available.

I was temporarily fixated on the fact that I was not doing what she wanted me to do, but my brothers helped me realize that the color of the casket wouldn't matter to Mom. She had only been trying to ensure that we wouldn't be paying for it. We moved on and chose a blue casket with a pale pink satin liner, agreeing Mom would like it. I let the funeral director know I would be bringing her clothing by on Monday after my meeting with Reverend Pierce.

Once we finished our business with the funeral director, we went to pick out Mom's flowers. We knew she loved pink carnations, pink roses, and white lilies, so those were our obvious choices. Once that task was completed, we finalized who would be serving as pallbearers (under Nicholas' direction), and realized there was nothing else we could do until after I met with the priest.

A meeting was scheduled with Reverend Pierce and Tom Peters, Mom's choice for officiant, for Monday morning to discuss the funeral. My brothers were not available to attend that meeting with me, so I let everyone know that I would call as soon as I had finalized details with the priest; once that was done, we would put together a to-do list. Lynn planned to join me so I wouldn't be by myself. Then Daniel adjusted his schedule for the same reason.

This planning was easy. We knew Mom would want a full Mass. We just needed to select readings and scriptures to be included in the service. I also needed them to review the order of service I had prepared to be included as part of the obituary. We had many non-Catholic family and friends, and I wanted them to be able to follow along with what was happening during the service.

Next, we needed to choose the music the church choir would be singing. Again, this was an easy task. Mom loved the song "On Angels' Wings," so that was a must. Her beloved "Holy, Holy, Holy" had been a great source of comfort during her final days, so it was included as well. The offertory hymn would be "Be Not Afraid" because she had experienced many moments of fear. "Joyful, Joyful We Adore Thee" and "Song of Farewell" were chosen as the final two selections because I knew she had liked them so well.

During our meeting, we learned that the food for repasts held at the Immaculate Conception Church was catered by Guido's. Without hesitation, we agreed to hold Mom's repast at the church. Guido's was Mom's number one choice for carryout, and we knew she'd be pleased with the idea of this restaurant catering her repast. She had trusted Guido's with the repasts for both John's and Lewis' funerals, so this was a no-brainer for us. I could sense her smiling at the thought of being honored by her beloved church.

After discussing calling hours, and Reverend Pierce's stating that he planned to come to offer a word of prayer during the same, our meeting was over. After taking Mom's burial clothes to the funeral home, Daniel, Lynn, and I grabbed some lunch to go and headed back to Mom's house to discuss what else was left to be done, and by whom.

The final order of business involved assigning the readings. When choosing people to do the readings, I tried to secure representation from the households of each of Mom's children. Nicholas and I agreed to represent our households because our kids did not feel they'd be able to stand before the congregation and do the readings. Don's and Lewis' daughters, Leigh and Veda, represented their households. Daniel had no children and chose not to do a reading.

Finally, the programs were ready for printing. Although none of us liked the photo we chose for the obituary, Mom had loved it. My son-in-law, Bill, offered to handle the printing of the programs, and I knew I could trust him one hundred percent to ensure the finished product would be acceptable to my scrutinizing eye. He did not disappoint.

On Tuesday, May 8, my brothers and I, along with our significant others, met at Mom's for lunch. Nicholas' company had sent a meal over, and it was nice to be able to sit and relax before taking on the events that were about to occur.

There was a steady stream of visitors during Mom's calling hours. People shared their stories, good and bad, of their experiences with our mom. Everyone commented on how beautiful Mom looked in her dress. She would have loved hearing that. She lay so peacefully, with her rosary and her mom's Bible softly resting in her hands.

As promised, Reverend Pierce came to offer words of prayer. When he peered into the casket he said, "She looks really good, like she is going to a wedding." Each time someone made a fuss over her appearance, I could imagine Mom smiling. That, in turn, made me smile.

When we left that night, I felt such a sense of dread thinking about Wednesday, the day of Mom's funeral. I said a silent prayer to God, asking for strength and endurance. I was tired and I was stressed. I wanted to feel confident that we would do a good job of honoring Mom and her wishes.

On Wednesday morning, George and I picked up Daniel and went to meet the rest of our immediate family at the funeral home for a private moment with Mom. The funeral was to be closed casket, so this would be our final time seeing Mom's face. When the last family member arrived, we walked into the funeral home and, one by one, said our final farewell to Mom. We then proceeded to the church for her service.

OBITUARY
Lottie Mae (Polk) Berry
Born to Earthly Life: April 2, 1928
Transition to Eternal Life: May 5, 2018

Lottie Mae (Polk) Berry was born to her late parents, Albert and Will Ella (Spires) Polk in Bentonia, Mississippi, where she was also raised. Upon graduating from high school, Lottie underwent special training to become an LPN. This career turned out not to be her cup of tea, and she quickly put her sights on other things.

Lottie met and later married the love of her life, John Willis Berry Jr. As the story is told, one day, while they were dating, John asked her to marry him. She responded, "Yes," and they proceeded to go to the courthouse to wed, to the dismay of their parents.

Lottie and John moved from Mississippi in the late 1940s, eventually migrating to Ohio where their children were raised and educated. The entire family converted to Catholicism, and they were all baptized as they became members of the Immaculate Conception Church in Ravenna, Ohio. Lottie was a devout Catholic whose faith was very important to her. It was that faith and the loving care of her family that sustained her during the final months of her life. She would often be seen praying to and speaking with God.

A retiree of the General Electric Company, Lottie held many careers during her lifetime, which included serving as a cook at Kent State University and at Howard Johnson's, and being a matron at the Portage County Jail. Many will tell you that she felt her greatest accomplishments were her children. She loved to boast of their successes and would often state, "Not one of them ever gave me a bit of trouble!"

Before becoming ill, Lottie enjoyed walking on the track at Kent State University, playing bingo, crocheting, working crossword puzzles, dining with friends, and grilling. She was grateful to her dear friends, Barbara and Eunice, who went out of their way to ensure that she was able to attend church and participate in desired activities for as long as was physically possible.

Lottie's main goal was to live to be ninety. No one knows exactly why it was so important to her, but it was. Praise God that her desire came to fruition, and that all of her children and some of her grandchildren were with her on her special day. We are so very grateful for that answered prayer!

In addition to her parents, Lottie was preceded in death by her one true love, John; her sons Lewis, John III, and Andrew; and her siblings Nettie B. (Polk) Berry, and Addie Polk. Lottie leaves behind many who will cherish her memory: children Don (Grace), LaBena (George) Fleming, Daniel, and Nicholas; grandchildren Veda, Richard, Thomas, Lucas, Anthony, Chris, Leigh, Lynn, Yvonne, Jennifer, and Paula; a host of great and great-great grandchildren; and nieces, nephews, and special cousins.

Mom, we feel nothing but gratitude for having you in our lives for as long as we did. You were a very strong, feisty woman who would do anything for your family. Your love knew no limits. You

were truly fierce, and we will miss you more than words can express.

Rest Well,
Your Children

For though I be absent in the flesh, yet am I with you in spirit, joying and beholding your order, and the steadfastness of your faith in Christ. Colossians 2:5

Chapter 22
Life Goes On

My brothers and I agreed that Mom would have been both proud and pleased with her send-off. She would have been even more proud of how we had worked so well together to ensure that all her wishes were honored. That, in turn, gave me a great sense of pride, and I'm fairly confident it did for my brothers as well. It was now time to handle business.

As the executor of Mom's estate, I contacted the life insurance company to have them instruct me regarding what process needed to be followed for payout and to ensure that they received a copy of Mom's death certificate. I also contacted her former employer to see if anyone would be entitled to her retirement fund and whether she'd had a death benefit with them. The funeral home notified the Social Security office of Mom's death.

Mom's bank account had been set up as payable on death, with my brothers and I listed as beneficiaries. Any funds remaining would be divided equally between the four of us. I contacted the bank and scheduled a time for us to meet with a representative at the bank. I wanted us all to be present at the same time so there would be no question that business had been conducted fairly. Earlier, when I had seen that Mom's death was imminent, we had met for dinner and I had provided everyone with a copy of Mom's bank statements for the few months leading up to her death. Although I felt my brothers trusted me, I wanted them to see that there had been no funny business going on regarding Mom's assets.

When we met with the bank representative, each of us was given a check for a portion of Mom's savings. We then went outside, said our farewells, and promised we would try to get together every couple of months. Mom had always served as the family glue. She was the common thread. Her home had been the meeting place for so many years. As we said our goodbyes, I wondered how long we would honor our promise to continue to get together. I was hopeful, yet doubtful.

As one final order of business, I needed to get the house transferred over to Daniel. This would also be easy, as Mom had already set it up to transfer to him on her death. We needed only to take Mom's death certificate to the auditor's office, along with appropriate identification, and fill out some paperwork. The entire process took less than an hour.

Lesson: Taking time to preplan is one of the greatest gifts you can give to your loved ones.

When we returned to Mom's—I mean, Daniel's house—he announced that he would immediately begin purging Mom's things and suggested that I take whatever I wanted. Photos had been previously divvied up. The house and all its furnishings were to go to Daniel if he wanted them. What he specifically wanted me to do was go through Mom's personal items. She had no jewelry of value that we knew of, so I just needed to go through her clothing.

The only clothing I was interested in keeping was a few coats I had given her over the last couple of years. I would come to take Mom shopping and find her wearing a coat that was either too large, too small, dirty, or torn. I'd literally end up giving her the coat off my back. Although I was larger than Mom, she liked wearing bulky clothing. As such, those coats would fit her just fine. As it turned out, the only coat I'd given her that was still wearable was a navy blue and beige Nautica jacket that I loved. Although it had several food spills on it, I was fairly certain I could have it cleaned, and it would be as good as new.

I had already gotten rid of items that were not fit to be worn and cleaned those that were. Since coming home from rehab, she had not worn any of those items, except a couple of pairs of sweatpants and sweaters. We bagged the remaining clothing, preparing it for pick-up by a local charity.

211

That was it. There was nothing else to do. All accounts had been settled. All debts had been paid. All necessary transfers had been made. I wondered what there was for me to do now. For the past year and a half, most of my life had revolved around Mom. I was Lottie's daughter, and one of her caregivers. Before that, I had been an employee of HWR. I had been a student, an employee, a wife, a mother. I had now reached a time in my life where I could be whatever I had chosen to be, but I hadn't the slightest idea of what that would be. I had always been defined by what I did but now had no idea what I was going to do. I was still a wife, mother, and nana, but what else?

As things began to settle down, I realized that Mother's Day was fast approaching. This would be my first Mother's Day without my mom. Was I supposed to celebrate it? I didn't want anyone to ask me what I wanted because I didn't want anything other than to pretend that day didn't exist. Perhaps I could just stay in bed all day. That's it . . . I'll just sleep the day away. Of course, that's not what happened.

Mother's Day was only eight days after Mom's death. That day, I got up and couldn't bring myself to go to church, which I had always done on Mother's Day in years past. I had enjoyed the special attention afforded to mothers on their day. I had enjoyed wearing corsages and when our pastor asked all mothers to stand so they could be acknowledged. I had enjoyed everyone approaching me and wishing me a Happy Mother's Day. Not this time. I did not want to be reminded that my mom was gone. I was fully aware, but I didn't want to think about it.

I could tell George was anxious, not knowing what to say or do. As was our usual, we got up and made the bed. He then walked to my side, kissed me, and asked if I'd like him to make breakfast or take me out for breakfast. I told him no but thanked him for the offer. He knew me well enough not to push. I lingered upstairs a little longer than usual, as I didn't want to have to make small talk while he ate breakfast. I'm sure he was relieved as well, not knowing what to say or how to say it.

I finally went downstairs and made myself a cup of coffee using the Keurig. George looked up from the newspaper. "Do you need anything? Is there anything I can do for you?" he asked. I thanked him for his offer; I was fine and just needed alone time today. He understood and complied, looking somewhat relieved but sad at the same time.

I sat at the table trying to read the newspaper, but my eyes kept welling up with tears. I received calls from Lynn and Yvonne wishing me a Happy Mother's Day and asking how I was. "Sad," I replied to each of them. I could tell they were sad for me. They tried to make small talk but eventually said their goodbyes and said they'd speak with me later. I did not want any company, so they would have to choose another day to bring their gifts to me.

I couldn't control my thoughts or my tears. I kept thinking of Mom and the fact that this was the first time I could not call her or see her on Mother's Day. This was the first of many firsts to come. The tears flowed freely now, as I saw George peer through the French doors that separated the living and family rooms. He came in, gave me a big hug, and said, "I know it's tough, and it's going to be tough for a while. It's going to take time." Time for what? I thought.

George's mom had died several years earlier as the result of a heart attack, so he knew what it felt like to lose a mom. What he hadn't experienced was being a caregiver for his mom. He hadn't had the gift of forming that special bond that I felt could only be formed when you spend a great deal of intimate time with someone who is dying. I felt Mom and I had a soul bond which he'd not had with his mom. He understood . . . but he didn't.

Because journaling had become a source of comfort for me of late, I decided to try to write what I was feeling.

Dear Mom,

Happy Mother's Day! Although I knew I would be sad today, my first Mother's Day without your physical presence, I was not expecting the flood of memories that have come. Initially, my eyes welled with

213

tears when I realized I couldn't call you. I could almost hear your voice saying, "LaBena, that's enough!"

The reality is I have been mourning your loss since dementia reared its ugly head more than ten years ago. The mom I knew was being slowly taken away from me. Surprisingly, glimpses of the old Lottie would show up now and then over the last couple of months. Along with those glimpses came some beautiful, tender moments. There were also some not-so-beautiful moments, to which your caregiver could attest.

So, Mom, when I feel the tears begin to flow, I am going to choose to remember:

... How we honored your wishes and gave you the send-off you desired. We may not have agreed on everything, but we never bickered. We realized it was all about you, and we did it your way.

... How we worked together to ensure you were able to return to your home and did everything in our power to ensure you had all that you needed. Again, no bickering or disagreements ensued. Everything was done with your desires in mind.

... How your eyes would light up every time Daniel entered the room. As your primary caregiver, he caught the brunt of your discontent over the years. It was beautiful to see the tender moments between the two of you, especially over the last two months of your life. I am grateful he was able to experience that relationship and have those special memories of you.

... How the caregiver would call me when you refused needed medications. Sometimes I could coax you into taking them, but most of the time I could not. I would call Don and he would drop whatever he was doing to go administer your meds. You always took them for him! I later found out that he would threaten to send you to a nursing home if you didn't. Shame!

... How Nicholas would stroke your forehead gently and you would relax. Whenever I did it you would say, "You can stop rubbing my head now." He always was your favorite!

... How I would come to visit, and you'd say, "Lady, get the hell out of my room!" I would come closer and put my face very close to yours and you would recognize me. I treasure the time you burst out laughing after you recognized me. That warmed my heart.

... How during our many lunches together, you would always have something to say about the people going through the buffet at your Evergreen Buffet. "Look at all that food that old fat thing is putting on his plate." Or perhaps it would be, "They could have at least tried to look decent. I wonder who dressed them this morning." I would always ask you to stop staring and you'd respond that you weren't staring, you were just looking. You'd always complain that the food was cold, even if it was steaming. You would also wrap eggrolls in napkins and slip them into your purse, even though you were not supposed to take food outside of the restaurant. No one would dare approach you to tell you that.

... How I would share my most recent pictures of Stinky Butt, which was one of your loving nicknames for Ann. You always asked about her and loved it when she joined us for lunch or came to visit you.

... How you loved unconditionally. Mom, you forgave the unforgivable. If anyone wronged you and chose to make amends, you allowed them to do so. Your dementia oftentimes made it very difficult to be around you, and people drifted away. However, if they returned, you always made them feel loved. You held no grudges. You were just happy to see them today.

... How you fought so very hard to see your ninetieth birthday and, by the grace of God, you did. You were ninety years and thirty-three days old when you went to be with God.

... How my dear friend Lena brought you flowers and candy for your birthday and you asked us to sing "Happy Birthday" to you. You also told us to "be friends forever."

... How you would incessantly call out to your cousins, Dank, Lucky, and Biney, a couple of weeks before your death. I think I began calling their names in my sleep.

215

... How you would think I was your sister, Nettie B. "Nettie B. Come up here," you would say. Once I'd get to the room, you'd always ask me what took me so long. One moment you'd be talking to me as if I were your sister, and the next you'd tell me to stop responding when you were calling your sister. Those were my favorite moments.

... How you would eat next to nothing throughout the day but suddenly develop an appetite when Daniel came in from work. Sorry, Nicholas, I think Daniel became her new favorite.

... How I would catch macho Daniel gently stroking your face or your hand when he would enter or exit the room. The devotion he showed to you was like none I'd ever seen. The bond the two of you formed was priceless.

... How you began having "visits" from those who'd passed on. Those visits seemed to comfort you. I specifically remember you turning your head towards the wall and saying, "I see Lewis. He's smiling." He died nine months before you, and his presence gave you some peace. You had been fighting for so long.

... How I was blessed to hear you say, "I love you always" for the last time on the Friday before Easter. It had been a while since I'd heard those words, so I cherished hearing them that day.

... How Daniel was at your bedside at 12:05 a.m. on May 5 when you took your last breath.

... How we, your children, honored you in life and death. I am so proud of us, and I am sure you are bragging about us up there in heaven, just like you did on earth!

Of course, the tears are flowing full force now, but it's okay. You are my mom, and I can cry if I want to. But I promise they are tears of joy as well as sadness. I miss you, but I am so happy you are no longer in pain and are in the arms of God. Your family will be fine. We will take care of each other just as you took care of us, for as long as you were able.

Chapter 23
A Year of Firsts

July would bring the first pleasant event since the death of my mom. It had always been a special month to me, with many birthdays (Yvonne, my dad, and me) and wedding anniversaries (Lynn and me). Now we would be adding another celebration: the wedding of Yvonne and my future son-in-law, Carl.

I felt guilty as I thought back to Mom's final months, when I would pray that she wouldn't die before or around the wedding, which was to be a destination wedding in Cancun, Mexico. If she died close to the wedding date of July 29, there would be no way I would go to the wedding that I had been looking forward to with great excitement. Would George go? He'd have to go. I was his wife and would need his support, but there is absolutely no way I'd allow him to miss his daughter's wedding.

What about Lena and her husband? Would they go to the wedding, or stay and support me? They had already paid for their trip. Was it even fair of me to consider the idea of their staying behind, knowing they would not receive a refund? If everyone close to me went to the wedding, who would be around to support me? Then the guilt had struck. Had I tried to negotiate a plan for when Mom would die? Why was it that I felt a bit of relief when Mom had died in May? In one moment, I had thought, I won't have to worry about Mom dying while I'm out of the country. Awful!

Lesson: You are human, with human thoughts and feelings. Don't feel guilty for feeling relief. Your loved one would not want that for you, and it serves no useful purpose.

The reality was that I would feel guilty many times in the upcoming months. I felt guilty anytime I wasn't sad, or whenever I laughed or found joy in something . . . anything. I felt guilty if I didn't think about how many days it had been since Mom had died, and if I didn't feel I was grieving long and hard enough. I felt guilty when I went to Yvonne's wedding and enjoyed myself instead of sitting and feeling sad. Guilty, guilty, guilty!

November 2018

It had been six months since Mom's death, and to say they were challenging would be an understatement. I was still attempting to find my flow. I had spent so much of whatever free time I'd had tending to Mom's needs that there was no time to figure out what was next for me. I went from working since the age of twelve to retiring at age sixty-two to immediately becoming a caregiver for my mom. I hadn't had time to figure out what I wanted my life to look like.

My brothers and I met only once for lunch since Mom's death. We asked how each other were doing and shared updates about our families, but beyond that, the conversation seemed awkward. Mom had been the center of our conversations for years. Now that she was gone, it seemed like we didn't have much to talk about. We were so different. We loved each other, but from a distance. That made me so sad.

Daniel rarely, if ever, allowed us to take him grocery shopping. He was able to get everything he needed either online or by riding his bike to the store. I believe the only reason he allowed us to take him in the past was because we were already going with Mom. He had always been independent, and now he was becoming more independent instead of the other way around. It's funny to consider how your world revolves around people, but at some point, they no longer need you. My sense of self was rapidly being lost in the process.

I have an amazing husband who held me together when I thought it would be impossible. I needed him in so many ways, but felt that although he loved and wanted me, he didn't *need* me. My girls didn't *need* me; they both had husbands who met whatever needs they had. I wanted to be needed and realized that no one needed me. I think I had, in the past, been defining myself by what I was able to do and be for others. Now, in my mind, there were no "others" who needed me to do anything for them.

To take my mind off everything, I began to plan Thanksgiving dinner. I had hosted dinner for more than fifteen years when Mom was no longer able to host. As a formality, I started making calls to see how many people would be in attendance this year. In the past, we always had Mom, Daniel, Lewis, Nicholas, his daughters, their significant others, and usually a few of George's family members.

When I called Nicholas, he seemed uneasy as he spoke about how far away I lived. I'd been living in the same general vicinity for over thirty years. Now I lived far away? I said, "You're not coming for Thanksgiving, are you?" He responded, "No." He would be joining his girlfriend and her family for the day. That meant his daughters wouldn't be coming either.

He then let me know that he had spoken with Daniel, offering to drive him to my home if he chose to come for Thanksgiving. When he said Daniel declined, I was not surprised. If Daniel didn't want us to drive him to the grocery store, he certainly wouldn't allow someone to drive him from Ravenna to Richmond Heights for Thanksgiving dinner. Daniel wanted to stay home and relax.

As I visualized my guest list diminish, I became sadder with each decrease. Yvonne and her new husband were starting their tradition of hosting Thanksgiving for their moms, siblings, and a few friends. I was happy they had their new tradition; however, I was sad for me. I knew Lynn, Bill, and Ann would come because, thankfully, they always came. My Thanksgiving was forever changed.

People had come to my home because Mom came. This would be my first Thanksgiving without my mom. Why did no one else realize how important it was for me to have them come? Why didn't they realize how much I needed their support? Couldn't they give me this holiday that's always been so important to me? How dare they do this to me?

How selfish of me! Despite my trying to make this about me, it was not just about me. All of us had experienced a loss. Lottie wasn't only my mom. I wasn't the only one who had loved and lost her. Just as I felt the need for things and traditions to remain as normal and same as possible, others felt the need to change and create. I went from being angry for people breaking my tradition to honoring their needs for something new.

Lesson: People grieve in their own way. Don't judge others because their method of survival is different from yours.

Thanksgiving was sad. I was sad, so everyone else was too. We went through the motions, but it wasn't the same; even the food tasted different. Something was missing. Everyone pretended to be jolly, probably attempting to ensure I wouldn't be caught up in my sorrow, but their eyes couldn't lie. I wanted it to be over, yet I knew that the next day we would just start moving toward another sad holiday: Christmas.

Christmas 2018

Holiday decorating had always given me joy. I loved making decorations, and I enjoyed purchasing them. I loved the praise I received when people admired my home décor. Because I loved shopping for Christmas gifts, I'd be one of those persons who would be out shopping on Christmas Eve, not because I'd forgotten to purchase something but because it was the one time of year that I enjoyed being in the hustle and bustle.

I loved the holiday music and how nice everyone was . . . or pretended to be. I would hope for light snow and hum "White Christmas" as I strolled from one store to another, not looking for anything. I would take my time admiring the beauty that was all around me. Occasionally, I would even reflect upon the reason for the season and send a silent thank you to God for the gift of His Son.

This year was different. I decorated the house, but something seemed to be missing. I'd frequently go out and purchase more decorations, only to be dissatisfied and think there was still something missing. No matter how many decorations I purchased and put up, something was missing. I didn't hope for light snow or hum "White Christmas." I didn't enjoy being amid the Christmas crowds and was irritated by the jovial attitudes of others, but I kept shopping. Something was missing.

On Christmas morning, George and I opened our gifts as we'd always done. His family alternated who would host Christmas brunch each year and, thankfully, it was my sister-in-law Marie's turn this year. I didn't want to go, but I did. We later went to the home of Nicholas' daughter for Christmas dinner. I didn't want to go, but I did.

I kept telling myself that something was missing, but it was not something but *someone* who was missing. I was missing my mom during the holidays. They just weren't the same without her and I wanted the holidays to be the same. I could feel our family beginning to pull apart without my mom—our glue—and I didn't like the way it felt.

Mother's Day 2019

On Mom's April 2 birthday, I went and placed silk pink carnations on her grave, staying long enough only to let her know how much I missed her. I told her I was happy she was no longer in pain and that she had been able to reunite with the loved ones she had missed so much.

This visit wasn't the painful chore I'd expected it to be, and I wasn't sad! Additionally, I didn't feel guilty for not feeling sad. This was only my second visit, having been there when they finally placed the headstone she had purchased the November before her death. My brothers and I had met to see how the stone looked on her grave. I remember Nicholas kidding that we add "Badass" to the tombstone. At least I think he was kidding.

221

I did not go to the cemetery on Cinco de Mayo, the anniversary of Mom's death, as I had planned. I had considered pouring a bottle of Miller High Life on her grave because she had loved it so much. I reconsidered, thinking that would be more sacrilegious than a tribute. She would be appalled if I'd desecrated the grounds of her beloved church cemetery.

I decided that it was time for me to stop being so hung up on Mom's death and try to begin truly honoring her life. It was funny of me to think that I had control over such a thing, but I knew that Mom would want me to move forward instead of staying stuck in my grief. I would do my best, I thought, as I told Mom that I loved her and said I'd have a Miller in her honor. I despise beer!

As Mother's Day approached, Lynn called to ask if I planned to go to the cemetery. "Yes," I responded. "I want to go with you," she'd replied. I was surprised, but I don't know why. I skipped church again, not yet ready to participate in the Mother's Day recognition, and made plans to pick up Lynn and drive to St. Mary's Cemetery. George stated that he'd planned to go with me but was opting out to allow Lynn and me some mother and daughter bonding time.

When I arrived at Lynn's home and rang the bell, Bill met me at the door and gave me a strong, long hug. Ann then approached me with a bag holding my Mother's Day gift, a diffuser with multiple scented oils, as Bill presented me with a bottle of ice wine. I knew I'd enjoy both gifts later! As Lynn came to the door, Ann donned her jacket as well. I asked where she was going, and she said, "I'm going with you, Nana, so you won't be sad." My heart leapt.

We didn't talk much on the way to the cemetery. Once we arrived, I made my usual stops, beginning with my brother Andrew's grave. Ann wanted to know all about him: How old was he when he died? What did he die of? Were you sad? These were just a few of the questions she asked. She then became fascinated by the many tombstones and went on a quest to find someone who had lived to be one hundred. St. Mary's is a small cemetery, with every inch of it visible from any given vantage point and only one road into and out of it, so we didn't blink when Ann said she would walk to the next grave.

Lynn and Ann walked together, Ann reading tombstones along the way, as I drove to my brother John's grave. John, Lewis, and Mom's graves were within a few steps of each other, so further driving was not necessary. When Ann reached my mom's headstone, she hugged it as she smiled broadly. I don't know what I had expected her to do, but that was certainly a surprise. She then went to John's and Lewis' graves, reading their stones as I placed new silk flowers near Mom's headstone where the ones I'd placed on her birthday, still immaculate, lay. I remember thinking that the groundskeepers took excellent care of the cemetery.

I looked up and noticed that Ann had gone to the mausoleum and was reading the various inscriptions. Suddenly she yelled loudly, "Nana, I found one! This guy was one hundred years old when he died." I smiled as I looked at my mom's headstone and said, "And you lived to be ninety. I love you always."

Lesson: Honoring someone in life, as well as honoring their life, is far more important than mourning their death.

O sing unto the Lord a new song: sing unto the Lord all the earth.
Psalms 96:1

Appendix

For information about Alzheimer's disease and other dementias, including facts and figures, symptoms, stages, resources, etc., contact the Alzheimer's Association at https://www.alz.org/

For a good resource on patient rights, Medicare coverage, and to access helpful tools for comparing nursing homes/SNFs, visit Medicare at https://www.medicare.gov/

To learn more about the hospice services provided by the organizations mentioned in this book, please visit:

Crossroads Hospice & Palliative Care:
https://www.crossroadshospice.com/

Hospice of the Western Reserve: https://www.hospicewr.org/

For more information about other medical conditions mentioned in this book, I consulted:

C. diff (*Clostridioides difficile*): https://www.webmd.com/
Hyperparathyroidism: https://www.parathyroid.com/
Sepsis: https://www.healthline.com/
Spinal stenosis: https://www.wikipedia.org/

LaBena's Fried Green Tomatoes

Ingredients

4 large green tomatoes
2 eggs
2 tablespoons of milk
2 cups of flour, divided (1 cup may be replaced with breadcrumbs
or cornmeal)
1 teaspoon of seasoned salt
Salt and pepper
Cooking oil

Instructions

Wash tomatoes and cut into 1/2-inch slices, discarding the ends.

Lightly sprinkle both sides of each slice with salt and pepper.

Prepare the dipping station. First, place one cup of unseasoned
flour on a plate or in a gallon-sized storage bag. Next, beat the eggs
and milk together in a bowl. Mix the remaining cup of flour,
breadcrumbs, or cornmeal with seasoned salt on a second plate or in a
second gallon-sized storage bag.
In the bottom of a large skillet, heat 1/2-inch of oil over medium
heat.
Flour each slice with unseasoned flour, dip it in egg mixture, and
then coat with seasoned flour, breadcrumbs, or cornmeal. Place in
heated oil, frying in batches so as not to crowd the skillet. Once one side
is golden brown, flip and brown the other side. Remove from skillet and
place on a paper towel to drain.

Enjoy!

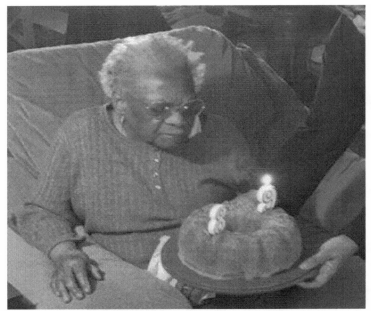

Lottie Mae Berry on her 89th Birthday. How quickly things changed!

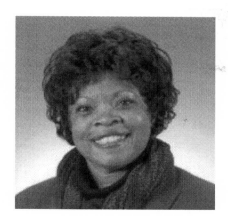

LaBena Fleming

LaBena Fleming was born in Detroit, Michigan, raised in Ravenna, Ohio, and presently resides in Richmond Heights, Ohio with her husband. LaBena received her bachelor's degree in human resources development from Notre Dame College of Ohio. She went on to earn master's degrees in elementary education and educational administration from Ursuline College in Pepper Pike, Ohio. A former insurance industry professional, elementary school teacher/administrator, and community education and outreach coordinator for an organ and tissue procurement organization, LaBena recently retired from her position as Provider Relations Manager/Community Outreach and Education Coordinator with Hospice of the Western Reserve. She served as one of her mother's primary caregivers and currently enjoys spending time with her husband, daughters, and granddaughter, public speaking, gardening, traveling, reading, and of course, writing.

Although she has always dabbled in writing, having written multiple poems and freelancing for a few greeting card companies, *I Love You Always* is her first book.

Made in the USA
Middletown, DE
21 July 2020

13368982R00144